Medicare Meets
Mephistopheles

Medicare Meets
Mephistopheles

DAVID A. HYMAN

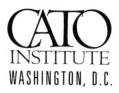

CATO
INSTITUTE
WASHINGTON, D.C.

Library of Congress Cataloging-in-Publication Data

Hyman, David Prof.
    Medicare meets Mephistopheles / David A. Hyman.
        p. cm.
    Includes bibliographical references.
    ISBN 1-930865-90-2 (cloth : alk. paper) — ISBN 1-930865-92-9 (alk. paper)   1. Medicare—United States—Popular works.   I. Title.

RA395.A3H96 2006
368.4'2600973—dc22   2006049565

Cover design by Jon Meyers.
Printed in the United States of America.

CATO INSTITUTE
1000 Massachusetts Ave., N.W.
Washington, D.C. 20001
www.cato.org

To Karen, Nathan, Benjamin, Rachel, and Eli

Difficile est saturam non scribere
(It is hard not to write satire.)
Juvenal, *Satires, I*

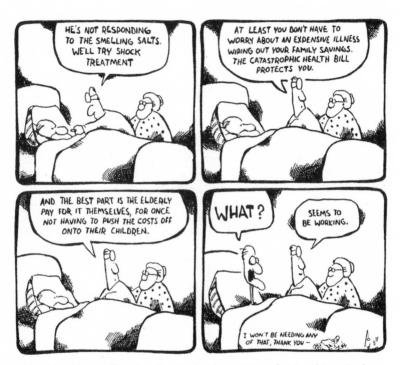

Contents

PART II — EPILOGUE

Foreword

I was about 22 years old when Medicare was first established in 1965, and to this day I remember my initial reaction to it. Think of two ways in which a group of 10 teenagers can drink soda at a luncheon counter. One is to get a large pitcher and have 10 thirsty kids each use a straw to take out what he or she wants. The second is to divide the soda into glasses, and assign them one to a person. Let there be 10 pints and each teenager's initial entitlement is one pint either way. The patterns of consumption of the soda will not be the same in these two arrangements. Even if by some miracle each person gets the same amount of soda in the two configurations (which they won't), we can be 100 percent confident that the soda will be more rapidly consumed when all 10 teenagers slurp their soft drink from the common pitcher. Consumption rates will slow markedly if each has his or her own glass, for slow sipping now results in greater satisfaction, not a reduction in individual share.

So why use this example in an introduction to David Hyman's *Medicare Meets Mephistopheles?* The tragedy of the commons arises because of a weak system of property rights to a given resource. Accordingly, the purpose of the law is to create some strong system of property rights that reduces the tendency to overconsume. Medicare, alas, works inexorably in the opposite direction, to create its own man-made tragedy of the commons. The control over health care resources is not a common by nature. Each individual owns exclusively his own person and wealth, and can freely trade something he has for something he desires more. Unfortunately, Medicare does not facilitate voluntary trade, but throttles it, producing the very risk of inequitable overconsumption that sound systems of law seek to avoid.

And so we must decide whether to laugh or to cry in the face of this multi-trillion-dollar mistake that encapsulates all that is wrong with the modern social welfare state. The Great Society worked overtime to encourage all takers to consume as much medical care as possible—but always at the expense of others. Far from strengthening private decisions and market institutions, it built a bewildering system whose massive cross-subsidies become apparent only with the passage of time. Yet once these are revealed, they generate widespread political conflict between those who want to keep or expand subsidies, on the one side, and those who want to remove or limit them, on the other. We created, as it were, an enormous pool of soda into which a vast armada may sink its straws.

Set against this stark backdrop, it becomes painfully clear why David Hyman invokes Juvenal as his muse and satire as his form of expression. *Medicare Meets Mephistopheles* evokes, of course, the Faustian image of the bargain that a hapless Faust made with the devil. But at least Faust had the excuse of falling in love with Gretchen to explain why he was prepared to mortgage his eternal future for the sake of his current pleasure. Learned psychologists might question the rationality of any person who would make a pact with the devil that works to his lifetime disadvantage.

There is, however, no need to question the rationality of the first generation of Medicare recipients. As Hyman never lets us forget, beneath Medicare's communitarian patina lies a program that thrives largely because it allows each generation to mortgage the future of the *next* generation. The communitarian rhetoric that launched Medicare masks its selfish underbelly. It is therefore entirely appropriate for Hyman to continue with the metaphor by grouping the consequences of Medicare under two headings: the seven deadly sins and the two lost virtues. To remind nonbelievers, these sins are avarice, gluttony, envy, sloth, lust, anger, and vanity. Our lost virtues are thrift and truthfulness.

As Hyman demonstrates, it is at once ironic and predictable that lofty communitarian aspirations have led to such anti-communitarian results. With stakes so high under Medicare, individual cunning and factional politics take center stage. The Medicare program imposes a heavy excise tax on young workers that acts as a barrier to entry into labor markets. But in the face of this burden, Medicare's determined defenders paint this massively redistributive and frequently regressive program as though it were a sacred intergenerational compact in which young and old alike benefit from their caring, if anonymous, relationships.

We are now in a position to understand why Hyman's distinctive contribution to satire succeeds. His basic hypothesis is that the Medicare program was created by Mephistopheles with the sole intention of bringing ruin on the United States. Concerned about the fate of his brainchild, Hyman's Most Exalted Satanic Majesty inquires of Underling Demon 666 about the fate of his program, only to receive an encouraging report of the success of his devilish master plan. The Underling starts from the simple premise that all human consequences of the Medicare program were intended by its Satanic sponsor. Hence every bit of bad news for the American people is good news for the devil. Unfortunately, Satan has much to crow about.

His first triumph lies in the original conceit behind the program. Lyndon Baines Johnson, a Texas populist, truly believed that one could redistribute wealth to a favored clientele without destroying wealth in the process. His defense of the program stressed how important it was to make sure that old people would not have to spend down their savings to care for their health. Nor would young people of the next generation have to watch their own incomes "eaten away" because of the obligation to care for their own parents. Both generations would win, simultaneously.

The secret to Johnson's marvelous sorcery was to stress only the gains from Medicare, barely stopping to ask who would pay the bill, or how large it would be. And, as is well understood, the devil lies in the details. On the first question, taxpayers and employers would pay the bills. In different guise they are the same family members who are supposed to receive protection against financial ruin under the program. It is easy to think you are rich if you look at the benefits that come into your left pocket, without taking note of the cash that has been taken from your right pocket.

But how much is paid? Happily for the devil, the great financial swap is not a wash, because the lesson of straws in soda holds true. Without direct financial restraint, people will consume more. So the original cost estimates that were politically pleasing were woefully wrong. By 1990, Satan had secured his pound of flesh: total hospital expenditures were more than six times those originally estimated in 1965. Of course, Medicare recipients were largely supportive or quiescent. Why not, when 75 percent of the money comes from other people? Cost-containment efforts failed to control spending but did achieve one of the devil's own objectives: they set patients against providers, and providers against each other, in an endless political struggle that saps the health care system to this very day.

One hope of Medicare's defenders was that quality and access would improve, even if at some high price. The latter goal was achieved, in part, for the senior citizens within the program. But the higher prices in the unregulated sector helped to increase the number of uninsured, reducing access especially among the young, the uneducated, and minority groups.

To make matters worse, quality measures are at best indifferent, for as Hyman notes, Mephistopheles seems to have had his way here as well. The political pressures were strong enough to prevent any solid measures of outcomes and productivity from being built into the system. The devil still claims that Medicare's low administrative costs have been a blessing, but that illusion has been achieved by the simple expedient of forcing higher compliance costs on providers, so as to keep some administrative costs off the federal budget. Satan knows that state monopolies can be at least as mischievous as private ones.

For the coup de grâce, consider whether we can find a way out of our present bind, which promises higher taxation and constant social dislocation. Reform is hard to come by because of the huge set of expectations and dependencies that have attached themselves to this system. The truly fiendish part is that Medicare's supporters made it very difficult to turn around to any less regulated system once we started down this road. What generation, having been pillaged by its elders, will fail to pillage its progeny? There are too many entrenched interest groups, and too much historical reliance on the system, to just shut it down. We have seen time and time again that economic expansions have helped the devil ward off a fundamental reexamination of the system. Mephistopheles should take great pride that with the passage of time it has become well nigh impossible to unravel and difficult to reform this bloated system. It would be easier to unscramble an omelet. Chances are good, Hyman concludes, that Mephistopheles will be able to maintain this system until ruin is upon us.

There is no point in continuing this dismal tale. The scribe of Mephistopheles has told it far better. So laugh, or cry, at his incisive account.

Richard A. Epstein
June 26, 2006

Preface

Medicare is the 800-ton gorilla of American health policy. Covering approximately 42 million (primarily elderly) Americans, it funnels almost $340 billion per year into the pockets of physicians, hospitals, clinical laboratories, home health agencies, physical therapists, social workers, pharmaceutical companies, and a veritable army of other health professionals. Medicare's administered pricing system can, whether by accident or design, shower largesse on particular regions, provider groups, and device manufacturers while starving others—with predictable consequences on the availability of the underlying goods and services. Medicare's regulatory requirements profoundly affect the institutional arrangements for the delivery of health care services to all Americans. Medicare's footprint is so large that its every move has spillover effects on the rest of the market.

Given Medicare's centrality to health care and health policy, it is not surprising that it has attracted considerable attention—including a 2003 conference at Washington and Lee University School of Law on "The Future of Medicare, Post–Great Society and Post–Plus Choice: Legal and Policy Issues." I was invited to speak at the conference, and the resulting papers were published in volume 60 of the *Washington and Lee Law Review*.

Michael Cannon of the Cato Institute (where I am an adjunct scholar) read my contribution to that volume and invited me to turn it into a short book, in the hope that my satirical take on Medicare would be of interest to a larger audience. Michael shepherded the book through the production process with considerable good humor—a trait in short supply when one is discussing Medicare inside the Beltway.

I appreciate the comments I received on this manuscript from various colleagues. All requested that I not name them because of the prospect of guilt by association. I also appreciate the comments I received when I presented the article at Washington and Lee University and the American Enterprise Institute.

This book was inspired by the works of a number of authors, including Stephen Vincent Benet, C. S. Lewis, Professor Uwe Reinhardt, and Mark Twain.[1] The "seed crystal" that precipitated the book was an offhand remark in an interview on PBS by Professor Reinhardt: "The devil systematically built our health insurance system that has the feature that when you're down on your luck [because] you're unemployed, you lose your insurance . . . only the devil could ever have invented such a system. Humans of goodwill would never do this."[2] Professor Reinhardt failed to consider that the devil might have a diversified portfolio of projects and would not limit his efforts to the employment-based health insurance system.

Introduction: The Memorandum

What follows is the demonic perspective on Medicare, contained in a document that appeared in my inbox. My secretary informed me that the document in question was delivered by a courier clothed in black and red, and driving a Lamborghini Diablo. The mailer bears an official-looking sticker, warning those who handle it that the envelope is made with asbestos fibers. The mailer also bears an extraordinary number of stamps, each bearing the likeness of Rodin's *Gates of Hell.* The document within the mailer is written on black parchment, reeks of brimstone, and singes the fingers of those unwary enough to handle it without insulated gloves. The words on each page glow red against the black parchment. The cover of the document is stamped with the legend "Abandon Hope All Ye Who Read Further."

The document, which is reproduced in chapter 1 of this book, purports to be a memo from a junior bureaucrat—Underling Demon 666, Deputy Assistant Special Coordinator for Accelerating Recruitment in the Department of Illness and Satanic Services—to the chief executive of his organization (Satan), reporting on the progress of their plans to use Medicare as a recruiting tool. The document was clearly important and deserved circulation to as wide an audience as possible—if only to alert the public of the depths to which opponents of Medicare would stoop to slime this sacred pillar of intergenerational equity.

Readers can judge for themselves the bona fides of the document and the merits of the observations contained therein. As for an appropriate disclaimer to the document itself, it is hard to improve on Mark Twain:

> PERSONS attempting to find a motive in this narrative will be prosecuted;
> persons attempting to find a moral in it will be banished;
> persons attempting to find a plot in it will be shot.[1]

PART I

MEDICARE AND THE SEVEN DEADLY SINS

1. Abandon Hope All Ye Who Read Further

To: His Most Exalted Satanic Majesty
         Lucifer, the Prince of Darkness
         King of the Damned
         Beelzebub
         His Nibs
         Master of the Nether Regions
         Scourge of the Self-Righteous
         Seventh Circle of Hell, Hell

From: Underling Demon 666
         Deputy Assistant Special Coordinator for Accelerating
            Recruitment (DASCAR)
         Department of Illness and Satanic Services (DISS)
         North American Division
         Washington, D.C.

Re: Market Share Report—United States of America

Per your request, I report herein on behalf of DISS on the progress of our attempts to corrupt the American Republic. Happily, our market share in the United States grows with every passing day. Our growth has been particularly precipitous since we repackaged our product in 1965.

As you know, the recipe we have used for centuries (avarice, gluttony, envy, sloth, lust, anger, and vanity—known collectively hereafter as the "seven deadly sins") has worked perfectly well in most of the known world. These sins were first cataloged by Pope Gregory "the Great,"[1] and have since been analyzed by such luminaries as St. Thomas Aquinas, Dante, Chaucer, and C. S. Lewis. They have also been featured in recent Hollywood movies and a wide array of advertisements. (My personal favorite is an ad for Las Vegas, your home away from home, that appeared in in-flight magazines. The ad featured a poker chip that bore the legend "Seven Deadly Sins, One Convenient Location.")

Unfortunately, Americans have proved unusually resistant to the charms of the seven deadly sins, even though your status as an American citizen should have been quite helpful in this regard. Through almost two centuries, Americans persisted in doing unto others as they would have done unto themselves, working hard and playing by the rules, staying in school, saving for a rainy day, going to church, donating to charities, volunteering their time to worthy causes, and generally behaving like goody two-shoes at every conceivable occasion. We have long had considerable success with our recruiting efforts among two groups of Americans: members of Congress and lawyers. (To be fair, we had a considerable advantage, given your status as the "King of Lawyers.")[2] However, these groups were unable to do serious damage as long as the rest of the population behaved themselves.

As such, it was a stroke of evil genius for your eminence to come up with the idea of creating a government program that would corrupt everything and everyone it touched, by incorporating all seven of the deadly sins, while simultaneously persuading the public that it included none of them.[3] The program works insidiously so that the citizenry is unaware of its evils until it is far too late. Indeed, they vigorously defend the program against

Demonic Citizenship

There is some dispute about your citizenship, as most nations claim that you are a citizen of their most hated enemy. However, my understanding is that you are a citizen of the United States of America. I refer your satanic majesty to the unfortunate incident in New Hampshire, where Daniel Webster asserted you were a foreign prince:

"Foreign?" said the stranger. "And who calls me a foreigner?"

"Well, I never yet heard of the dev—of your claiming American citizenship," said Dan'l Webster with surprise.

"And who with better right?" said the stranger, with one of his terrible smiles. "When the first wrong was done to the first Indian, I was there. When the first slaver put out for the Congo, I stood on her deck. Am I not in your books and stories and beliefs, from the first settlements on? Am I not spoken of, still, in every church in New England? 'Tis true the North claims me for a Southerner, and the South for a Northerner, but I am neither. I am . . . an . . . American."[4]

I also note that in a recent case, your citizenship was uncontested.[5]

all criticism, and, ironically enough, believe the program's critics are allied with us!

I refer, of course, to the Medicare program, whose every feature bears the distinctive stamp of your subtle genius. Chapter 2 provides some background on the Medicare program, how it came about, and where it is headed. Chapters 3–9 catalog how the Medicare program incorporates and reinforces the effects of each of the seven deadly sins. Chapter 10 outlines how Medicare further undermines two distinctively American virtues: thrift and truthfulness. Chapter 11 outlines a number of threats to our plans, and Chapter 12 offers a brief conclusion.

2. Medicare Overview

This chapter provides an overview of various salient features of Medicare, including its origins, structure, financing, and the like.

Medicare's Origins

President Lyndon B. Johnson signed the legislation establishing Medicare on July 20, 1965. To mark President Harry Truman's efforts to enact such a program 20 years earlier, President Johnson chose to sign the bill at the Truman library in Independence, Missouri, with President Truman at his side. A picture of the signing ceremony adorns my wall, to commemorate the launch of your most ambitious plan to destroy the American Republic. The photo is reproduced below for your reference.

Those present included various congressional leaders, including the person standing on the far right side of the picture, Representative Wilbur Mills. As the chairman of the House Ways and Means Committee, Mr. Mills shepherded the Medicare bill through Congress, and was the person most responsible for Medicare's basic design features.

Despite our best efforts, Mr. Mills was deeply concerned about the fiscal implications of making the government the primary payer for health care services for the elderly. Mills's fiscal conservatism and his commitment to budgetary restraint led him to design Medicare's financing in a way that forced policymakers to periodically confront the growing costs of the program.[1] We opposed this financing plan, out of the fear that early cost overruns

9

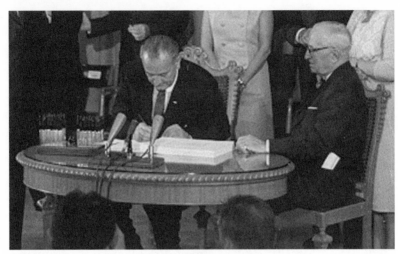

Courtesy Lyndon Baines Johnson Presidential Library.

would cause Congress to wise up and kill the program in its infancy. However, we were pleasantly surprised by the passivity of Congress and the American public in the face of a program that was dysfunctional from the get-go.

Such concerns were far from the mind of President Johnson when he signed the Medicare bill. Instead, his signing statement reflects the deeply moralistic overtones of his campaign for Medicare, and his hopes for the future:

> No longer will older Americans be denied the healing miracle of modern medicine. No longer will illness crush and destroy the savings they have so carefully put away over a lifetime so they might enjoy dignity in their later years. No longer will young families see their own incomes, and their own hopes, eaten away simply because they are carrying out their deep moral obligations to their parents, and to their uncles, and to their aunts. . . . No longer will this nation refuse the hand of justice to those who have given a lifetime of service and wisdom and labor to the progress of this progressive country.[2]

The Stripper and the Congressman

We rewarded Mills's attempts to frustrate our designs for the American Republic by luring him into an affair with a stripper from Argentina, Annabelle Battistella, whose stage name was Fanne Foxe, the Argentine Firecracker. In the early morning hours of October 7, 1974, Mills and Foxe were driving near the Tidal Basin in Washington, D.C. When the D.C. Park Police pulled over the car for speeding, Foxe attempted to flee the scene and jumped into the Tidal Basin. The incident attracted national publicity and Mills resigned as chairman of the House Ways and Means Committee two months later. Mills was reelected in 1974, but announced in 1976 that he would not seek reelection. Foxe continued working as a stripper, changing her stage name from "the Argentine Firecracker" to "the Tidal Basin Bombshell." She also wrote a book (which is available in our library) titled *The Stripper and the Congressman.*

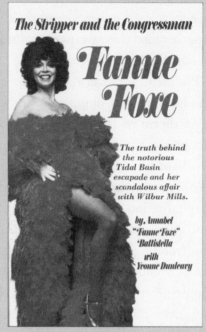

11

Of course, the irony is that President Johnson gave little thought to the long-term cost burdens imposed by the Medicare program. Yet, as you anticipated, these burdens fall disproportionately on working families—who now, in President Johnson's own words, "see their own incomes, and their own hopes eaten away," this time because they are paying the exorbitant taxes necessary to sustain the Medicare program.

President Johnson's optimism about the program notwithstanding, a better indicator of the long-term fiscal consequences of Medicare was the simple fact that President Truman was the first person to receive a Medicare card for hospitalization benefits. It is hard to make the case that ex-presidents are in need of any sort of subsidy from ordinary working Americans to pay for their hospitalization expenses—but that is exactly what Medicare did (and does). As if this reverse–Robin Hood scheme for hospitalization (robbing from the working poor to give to the wealthy) was not bad enough, President Truman also "doubled down" and simultaneously applied to enroll in the voluntary part of Medicare that covers physician treatment (supplementary medical insurance or SMI). There was no attempt to hide the reverse–Robin Hood scheme; the form that President Truman signed made it clear that the federal government "will pay half the cost of this insurance." Once again, it is hard to make the case that ex-presidents are in need of any sort of subsidy from ordinary working Americans to pay for the cost of seeing a physician—but that is exactly what Medicare did (and does). For your reference, I have included a copy of President Truman's application for SMI, which was witnessed by President Johnson after the signing ceremony.

This degree of candor about the subsidies created by the Medicare program is unusual. Proponents of reverse–Robin Hood schemes usually know better than to advertise the extent to which

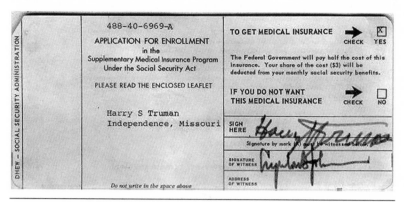

Courtesy Lyndon Baines Johnson Presidential Library.

the benefits received by upper-income beneficiaries come out of the pockets of lower-income taxpayers. Yet, Medicare's proponents were not embarrassed (as most people would have been) by this fact. Indeed, they actually celebrated the reverse–Robin Hood nature of the program, reasoning that it was only the first step toward having the federal government provide health insurance for the entire population (i.e., "universal coverage") through a system of "social insurance" where everyone pays for everyone else's health care coverage.[3]

Medicare Beneficiaries

Generally, Medicare is available for people age 65 or older, younger people with disabilities, and people with permanent kidney failure. Medicare currently provides health care coverage for approximately 42 million Americans, although this figure is expected to rise rapidly as the baby boom generation retires. Of course, as you anticipated, the population as a whole is not expected to increase as dramatically—meaning that the number

13

Figure 2-1
MEDICARE: MORE TAKING OUT, FEWER PUTTING IN

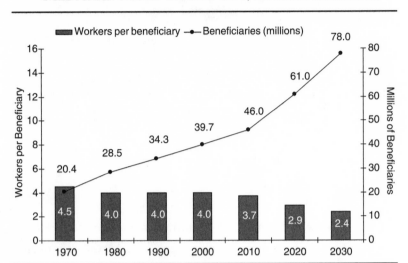

SOURCE: CMS Data Compendium, 2003; Annual Report of the Board of Trustees of the Federal Hospital Insurance and Federal Supplementary Medical Insurance Trust Funds, 2001, 2005.

of workers per beneficiary will drop substantially. Figure 2-1 shows how these two trends interact with each other.

These demographic mismatches create obvious challenges for financing Medicare—challenges that we are planning to exploit to our full advantage.

Medicare's Structure and Benefits

Medicare has four parts: Part A (hospitalization benefit), Part B (outpatient services), Part C (managed care), and Part D (pharmaceuticals).

As noted earlier, Parts A and B date to the beginning of the Medicare program. Part C was added to the program in 1997, as part of a balanced budget act (oh, the irony!), and is on its second incarnation. Part C was originally called Medicare + Choice, but Congress renamed it Medicare Advantage in 2003. Part D was enacted into law as part of the Medicare Prescription Drug Improvement and Modernization Act of 2003, also known as the Medicare Modernization Act, or MMA for short. Part D provided a preliminary prescription drug benefit (a drug discount card), with the full benefit package becoming available in January 2006.

Neither Part A nor Part B pays for all of a covered person's medical expenses, since there are various deductibles, copayments, and noncovered expenses. The most important exclusion is that Medicare does not cover long-term nursing care. Overall, Medicare pays for roughly 45 percent of the health care expenditures of its beneficiaries.[4]

Financing Medicare

Different parts of Medicare are financed in different ways, and each has different copayments and deductibles. Part A is almost entirely funded by a 2.9 percent tax imposed on all wages. Self-employed individuals pay the full tax of 2.9 percent directly, whereas 1.45 percent is withheld from the wages of employed individuals and the employer directly pays a matching amount. To be sure, the full burden of this tax is borne by the worker, regardless of how it is nominally split between the employer and employee—but it was yet another example of the extent of your evil genius to hide the true cost of the program from the chumps who are paying for it.

Of course, both the tax rate and the amount of wages subject to the Medicare tax have increased dramatically since the program was initiated in 1965. For high-wage workers, Medicare taxes can exceed the taxes imposed to keep Social Security (another of our programs) going.

Medicare beneficiaries with 40 or more quarters of Medicare-covered employment pay no premiums to receive benefits under Medicare Part A. People who are eligible for Medicare based on their age, but who do not have the necessary number of quarters of Medicare-covered employment may participate in Part A if they pay a hefty monthly premium. Beneficiaries who are hospitalized pay an initial deductible, plus copayments for all hospital days following day 60 within a benefit period.

Part B is financed with money allocated from general tax revenues and premiums paid by beneficiaries. All services provided pursuant to Part B are generally subject to a deductible and copayment, but certain medical services and related care are subject to special payment rules. Originally, the cost of Part B was evenly split between the government and the beneficiary. Consistent with our plan to use the Medicare program to destroy the fiscal solvency of the United States, we lobbied to have this ratio shifted to 75:25, with taxpaying citizens bearing the larger share and beneficiaries bearing the smaller share. We have ruthlessly demagogued any effort to change the ratio back to the original allocation.

Part C combines Parts A and B, and so its financing combines them as well. Part D is financed with a combination of premiums from beneficiaries, and substantial contributions from general tax revenues. However, Part D is an interesting hybrid, since low-income seniors pay lower premiums and have lower cost sharing to receive benefits.[5] In the past, Medicare beneficiaries could qualify for such treatment only if they were "dual eligibles"—that is, they were eligible for both Medicare and Medicaid. (As you recall, Medicaid is the medical insurance program for the poor that Medicare's opponents offered in 1965 as an alternative to our product. Rather than serve as a substitute, however, this similarly pernicious program[6] was bundled and enacted *alongside* our product.[7])

We have routinely opposed means testing of Medicare, on the grounds that it would undermine public support for the program. The MMA also introduced limited means testing for Part B, and we ultimately decided not to oppose that provision because the rest of the MMA helped advance our mission. We could also see the writing on the wall; the financial projections for Medicare had gotten so bad that even the Clinton administration seriously considered means testing. A strategic retreat on means testing for Part B also helped preclude a serious debate over means testing for Part A, where the adverse consequences for our plans would be much more severe. (This memo returns to means testing in chapter 11.)

Despite these variations, what Parts A–D have in common is that they are overwhelmingly (i.e., between 75 percent and 90 percent) financed by taxpayers who are not receiving benefits from the Medicare program. Figure 2-2 shows the distribution of the costs of Medicare.

As we had hoped, this perverse allocation of the costs of Medicare has not attracted much attention, since we positioned Medicare as a sacred intergenerational trust—effectively distracting almost everyone from the staggering amounts of money being spent. No one but the devil could ever come up with such a clever plan—let alone persuade the American public that this regressive financing structure was desirable!

Medicare's Administrative Structure

When it was created, Medicare was administered by the Social Security Administration. Although the SSA is still responsible for

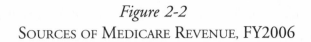

Figure 2-2
SOURCES OF MEDICARE REVENUE, FY2006

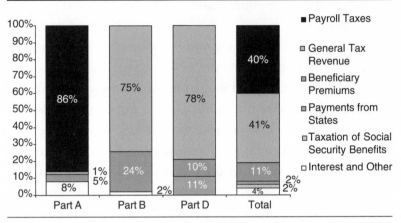

SOURCE: "Medicare Fact Sheet: Medicare Spending and Financing," Kaiser Family Foundation, April 2005, p. 2, http://www.kff.org/medicare/upload/7305.pdf.

enrolling beneficiaries and collecting Part B premiums, operational control of Medicare was transferred to the Health Care Financing Administration in 1977. HCFA was renamed the Centers for Medicare & Medicaid Services (CMS) in 2001.

Medicare purchases medical care from more than a million providers of goods and services, including hospitals, skilled nursing facilities, home health agencies, clinical laboratories, HMOs, medical equipment suppliers, and physicians. To do so, it processes over one billion fee-for-service claims per year, making it the nation's largest single purchaser of health care. At present, Medicare pays roughly 17 cents of every dollar spent on health care in the United States.[8] In terms of the supply side, Medicare is responsible for roughly 31 cents of every dollar received by U.S. hospitals, and 24 cents of every dollar spent on physician services.[9]

A Rose by Any Other Name?

The name change from HCFA to CMS took place on July 1, 2001. Health and Human Services Secretary Tommy Thompson explained that "to give the agency a new direction, a new spirit, it is necessary that we give it a new name—one that truly reflects the agency's vital mission to serve millions of Medicare and Medicaid beneficiaries across America."[10]

At a Federal Trade Commission–Department of Justice hearing on health care and competition, CMS Administrator Tom Scully, with tongue firmly in cheek, suggested that the administration had actually changed the name of HCFA to CMS because everyone hated HCFA and changing the name would confuse people:

> The fact is, the health care market . . . is extremely muted and extremely screwed up and it's largely because of my agency. For those of you who don't follow CMS, which used to be called HCFA, we changed the name because it was so well loved. I always say it's kind of like when Enron comes out of bankruptcy, they'll probably change their name. So, HCFA—Secretary Thompson and I decided to confuse everybody. We changed the name to CMS for a couple of years so people wouldn't realize we're actually HCFA. So far, it's worked reasonably well.[11]

Administrator Scully did not exaggerate the dislike for HCFA on Capitol Hill, where it is viewed as a "rigid, heavy-handed regulator, more eager to set prices than to encourage competition or reward efficient providers of care,"[12] and "the corner of the federal government that, perhaps more than any other, politicians loved to hate"[13] because it has "three times as many regulations as the [Internal Revenue Service, and] . . . is disliked by nearly everyone except its beneficiaries [because it is] too restrictive, requires too many forms to be filled out, [and] takes ages to reimburse claims."[14]

No one has been able to explain why the acronym is not CMMS. Perhaps CMMS was less euphonious or harder to pronounce than CMS? Or perhaps the CMS administrators didn't want to advertise their involvement with Medicaid, the less popular federal program underwriting health care services for the poor? Of course, since the early favorite for a new name was Medicare and Medicaid Agency, we should all be appreciative that we did not end up with MaMA running Medicare.

When Medicare was created in 1965, it paid hospitals based on the cost of the care they provided, and physicians based on their "usual, customary, and reasonable" charges—thus adopting the payment systems that prevailed in the private coverage market. This open-ended reimbursement system had the immediate and continuing inflationary consequences we had hoped for. Since we had designed Medicare so its payment system could be changed only by an act of Congress, it has been extraordinarily difficult to reform the Medicare program, no matter how dysfunctional the status quo—even as the private coverage market abandoned the health care financing and delivery models that prevail to this day in Medicare.

When the pathologies of this payment system became too much for even Congress to bear, it finally authorized several complex "administered pricing" schemes, which allowed Medicare to dictate prices to providers rather than the other way around. These administered pricing schemes took effect in 1983 (for hospitals) and 1992 (for physicians). Both marked modest improvements on the systems that prevailed previously, but thanks to our lobbying efforts, the new systems have sufficient pathologies that they help advance our plans as well.[15]

For hospitals and nursing homes, Medicare employs a prospective payment system (PPS). The system pays a set amount of money for each episode of care falling into a set "diagnosis-related group," or DRG, regardless of the actual amount of care used. These DRGs effectively cap the incentive for hospitals to "run up the bill" on any given admission, since hospitals make money only when their costs are less than the DRG payment. Conversely, they create some incentives to discharge patients "quicker and sicker," to "upcode" hospitalizations so they are paid in a higher-level DRG, and engage in a variety of other ways to game the system. The basic "vice" of the PPS is that it cannot mimic the price-setting function of a competitive market. As such, it is not a real impediment to our plans. The system also creates huge incentives for congressional meddling, as hospitals agitate for special treatment, and individual senators and representatives attempt to "tweak" the PPS to the advantage of favored institutions.

For physicians, Medicare uses the Resource-Based Relative Value Scale, a deliciously complex system, to set prices for each service. Services receive a weighted value based on the amount of physician work, practice expenses, and the cost of malpractice insurance. The relative value is then multiplied by a conversion factor to determine how much the provider should be paid. Like the PPS, the RBRVS system has a whole set of pathologies. Because the government is setting the price for every service, the RBRVS system has spawned a never-ending cycle of "rent seeking," controversy, and congressional meddling, as each specialty group agitates for a higher rate for their particular services. In this regard, it is no accident that health care is responsible for more spending on lobbying than any other industry—and has been so for some time.[16]

Remarkably enough, almost no one has asked why the form of price setting used by the government in other parts of procurement (competitive bidding) is effectively nonexistent in Medicare. Only in durable medical equipment is there significant reliance on competitive bidding, and even that was immensely controversial. As chapter 6 reflects, efforts to introduce competitive bidding into Part C foundered in response to vigorous local opposition, and the competitive bidding provisions in the MMA are not scheduled to commence until 2010. This "dessert first, spinach later" strategy was effective when Medicare was launched, and we expect it will continue to be effective right up until the apocalypse.

Quality of Care

When Medicare was created, the issue of quality was left to physicians and hospitals. Attempts to impose limited oversight in the early 1970s precipitated a major battle with those provider groups. There is more oversight of quality at the present time than there used to be, but that isn't saying much—and thankfully, what there is isn't particularly effective.[17]

There is, however, plenty of evidence on the quality of care delivered to Medicare beneficiaries, and I am proud to say the care is just what we had hoped for: highly mediocre overall, with some of it absolutely appalling. Medicare pays (and pays and pays . . .), but it gets every conceivable variety of quality problems: overuse, underuse, misuse, unexplained variations in treatment patterns, and outright errors. Numerous studies have quantified the magnitude of these quality problems—and I am pleased to tell you that not one of the studies blames us for the woes that beset Medicare and its beneficiaries. Instead, the list of villains includes defective incentives, poor information, inadequate monitoring, the state of medical science, noncompliant patients, incompetent providers, and everything else one could imagine. Of course, not all of these factors were our doing, but the way you designed Medicare exacerbates even the problems we did not create.

Because these studies typically focus on individual diseases and interventions, and there are so many of them, it is hard to cover the subject adequately under the space constraints you imposed. Instead, I will focus on a single recent study that gives a fair sense of the quality of care actually delivered to Medicare beneficiaries. This study focused on the quality of care delivered on a state-by-state basis for six different medical conditions (heart attack, breast cancer, diabetes, heart failure, pneumonia, and stroke) that affect large numbers of Medicare beneficiaries.[18] To evaluate the quality of care, the study used 24 measures for which there was a strong scientific basis. The theoretical goal for each measure was for 100 percent of qualifying Medicare beneficiaries to receive the intervention. In fact, depending on the measure, performance rates in the median state ranged from 24 percent to 99 percent. Median performance in the median state was 73 percent—which would receive a grade of C- in most places (except for law schools, where it would be a solid B). This study clearly shows that many Medicare beneficiaries are not receiving high-quality care. Yet Medicare keeps on paying, oblivious to that poor-quality care.

A distinct quality problem afflicting the Medicare program is the considerable regional variation in treatment patterns, with little or no evidence of benefit—and some evidence of harm! Consider death, which has allowed us to close so many open accounts. In theory, there should be little variation in the treatment patterns in the six months that precede death, since we have, by definition, controlled for the ultimate outcome. Yet, there are staggering disparities in the likelihood of dying in the hospital, how many days are spent in the hospital, how many days are spent in the intensive care unit, and the like, even when the Medicare beneficiary has been admitted to one of the "best" hospitals in the United States.[19] More generally, for many treatments, there are four- to sixfold variations in treatments rates, even in geographically contiguous locations.[20] Some regions even have distinctive "surgical signatures," where there are stable but highly variable region-specific idiosyncratic rates for surgical procedures.[21]

An angel might have hoped that quality of care would be better in places where Medicare spends more money, but we took care of that possibility as well. As one set of experts concluded, "Residents of high-spending regions received 60 percent more care but did not have lower mortality rates, better functional status, or higher satisfaction."[22] Instead of buying better care, more money just buys "more physician visits, more frequent use of specialist consultations, more frequent tests, and greater use of the hospital and intensive care unit."[23] We have done our job so well that one study found a negative correlation between quality and Medicare spending![24]

All of these problems are brought to you courtesy of Medicare's open-ended reimbursement system, where individual providers have virtually complete autonomy in their clinical decisions, and almost the only way a provider can get kicked out of the program is by committing a felony.

Administrative Oversight

Medicare's proponents routinely brag about its low administrative overhead. Of course, the figure is artificially low because Medicare has no marketing expenses, and it uses employers, the Internal Revenue Service, and the Social Security Administration to collect and process its premiums.[25] Despite these comparative advantages, the Medicare program has such inadequate financial controls that it hemorrhages money. Indeed, in a series of reports, the Office of the Inspector General for HHS concluded that roughly 7 percent of Medicare payments are "improper."[26] Although the Government Accountability Office and Office of the Inspector General routinely issue reports condemning particular financial shenanigans and labeling Medicare a "high-risk program," there has been only limited progress in bringing fiscal discipline to the program.[27] If anything, there is considerable evidence that Medicare's administrative expenses are too low for the program to be run properly—exactly the outcome we had hoped for.[28]

3. Avarice

Medicare promotes avarice among the 1.3 million providers that are collectively paid almost $340 billion per year for providing goods and services to Medicare beneficiaries. Indeed, it was only with avarice that we were able to get Medicare going, because many of these providers (especially physicians) were wary of the long-term consequences of inviting the federal government to become the major purchaser of health care services. Stated bluntly, Medicare was viewed as socialized medicine, and vigorously opposed for that reason.[1] The following cartoon exemplifies the degree of provider animosity we faced.

The American Medical Association fought long and hard against our efforts to enact Medicare, including one noteworthy episode involving our frequent adversary, Ronald Reagan. That episode is recounted in the following sidebar.

In any event, we were able to overcome provider opposition to our nefarious plans by appealing to their avarice with the prospect of staggering amounts of money—even as our actuaries were promising Congress that the Medicare program would be easily affordable.

We also told providers that we would never, ever interfere with the exercise of their professional judgment, or with beneficiary free choice. Indeed, the first two sentences in the original Medicare statute make those exact promises:

> Nothing in this title shall be construed to authorize any
> Federal officer or employee to exercise any supervision

or control over the practice of medicine or the manner in which medical services are provided, or over the selection, tenure, or compensation of any officer or employee of any institution, agency, or person providing health services; or to exercise any supervision or control over the administration or operation of any such institution, agency, or person. Any individual entitled to insurance benefits under this title may obtain health services from any institution, agency, or person qualified to participate under this title if such institution, agency, or person undertakes to provide him such services.

Of course, you broke both of those promises—but after all, you are the Prince of Darkness. Providers should have seen that one coming.

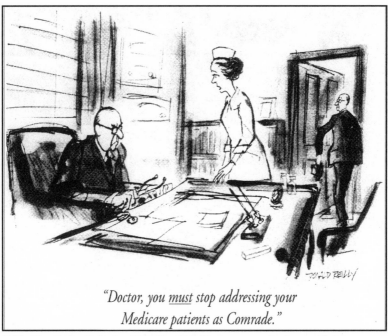

*"Doctor, you must stop addressing your
Medicare patients as Comrade."*

Operation Coffee Cup

In 1961, the AMA initiated Operation Coffee Cup, as part of its lobbying effort against Medicare. The wives of physicians were asked to invite their friends over for coffee and conversation, and they played a record provided by the AMA in which Ronald Reagan spoke out against socialized medicine. They then asked their friends to write letters to their congressmen, expressing their personal opposition to socialized medicine, and to the specific bill that Congress was considering in 1961.

Operation Coffee Cup was so successful, it delayed our timetable for the implementation of Medicare a full four years. I retrieved a copy of the record from our archives. To refresh your recollection about one of our more humiliating (albeit temporary) defeats, I have reproduced the cover and a short summary from the back of the album below.

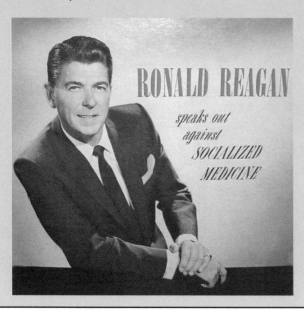

The Problem:
The legislative chips are down. In the next few
months Americans will decide whether or not this
nation wants socialized medicine . . . first for its
older citizens, soon for all its citizens. The pivotal
point in the campaign is a bill currently before Congress. The [bill] . . . is a proposal to finance medical
care for all persons on Social Security over 65, regardless of financial need, through the Social Security
tax mechanism. Proponents admit the bill is a "foot
in the door" for socialized medicine. Its eventual
effect—across-the-board, government medicine
for everyone!

Interestingly, this episode came to light almost 20 years
later, during the debate between then Governor Reagan and
President Carter. The debate was held one week before the
1980 election. When President Carter accused Governor
Reagan of opposing Medicare before its inception, Governor
Reagan responded, "There you go again." The audience
dissolved into laughter. President Carter had already gotten
into difficulty when he observed earlier in the debate that
he had consulted with his daughter Amy on arms control
strategy in preparation for the debate.[2] Many commentators
believe these two moments in the debate ensured President
Reagan's landslide election victory—positioning him to
label our allies in the Soviet Union as an "evil empire."

Medicare has resulted in extraordinary wealth for providers—not quite, as Samuel Johnson once put it, "beyond the dreams of avarice,"[3] but close. Yet, the whole point of avarice is that more than most is never quite enough, and providers ceaselessly agitate for increases in Medicare payments. As a concentrated special interest, providers have had considerable success in extracting ever-increasing sums from the federal fisc—in many instances convincing Congress to specify payment rates well in excess of those that would prevail in a free market.[4] As one former CMS administrator put it, "There are plenty of $400 toilet seats in the Medicare program because Medicare cannot deliver services to its beneficiaries without providers and because providers are major sources of campaign contributions in every congressional district in the nation."[5] Consistent with our larger goals, and as outlined in chapter 2, Medicare's compensation arrangements pay providers based on their inputs (procedures performed or time spent) and not their outputs (high-quality care actually delivered)—with predictable results on the quality and cost of care.[6]

Congress initially failed to appreciate how avarice would affect the Medicare program. When Medicare was enacted in 1965, a single provision prohibited making false statements to secure reimbursement. Matters did not remain in this pristine form for long, as the Medicare honeypot quickly attracted the more feloniously inclined members of the profession. In relatively short order, there developed a complicated interlocking array of health care-specific civil, criminal, and administrative anti-fraud laws and regulations enacted by the states and the federal government, along with multiple levels of investigative and enforcement agencies.[7] The following sidebar provides some background on how

Medicare Fraud and Abuse Laws: A Primer

Although a wide range of laws are potentially implicated by health care fraud, the three most significant provisions (anti-kickback, Stark, and false claims) are briefly outlined below.

Anti-Kickback

The anti-kickback statute was first enacted in 1972, and explicitly prohibited "kickbacks, bribes, or rebates" in connection with items or services for which payment could be made under Medicare.[8] For example, specialists and medical labs were prohibited from paying a general practitioner for sending business their way. No specific intent was required, and violation was a misdemeanor. The anti-kickback statute was substantially broadened in 1977 to include the solicitation or receipt of *any* remuneration, whether direct or indirect, overtly or covertly, in cash or in kind, in connection with items or services for which payment could be made under Medicare. Violation of the statute became a felony, subject to a maximum fine of $25,000 and imprisonment for up to five years. Various statutory and regulatory exceptions were created. Criminal prosecutions under the anti-kickback law have been relatively rare, and prosecutors have generally focused on the most egregious violations. Thus, the anti-kickback law provides fraud enforcers with a tool of tremendous power, but it is a tool that has, to date, received relatively limited use.

Self-Referral (Stark Amendments)

In 1989, Congress passed a limited prohibition on "self-referral" as part of a larger budget reconciliation act.⁹ This provision, which was inserted at the insistence of Rep. Fortney (Pete) Stark, by whose name it is commonly known (Stark I), prohibits physicians from referring Medicare patients to a clinical laboratory in which they hold a financial interest, and prohibits the clinical laboratory from billing for services performed as a result of such referrals. In 1993, Congress passed Stark II, which prohibits physicians from referring Medicare patients to 10 additional categories of providers in which the referring physician or a family member has a financial interest and prohibits those providers from billing for services performed as a result of such referrals. Because Representative Stark wanted to cover every conceivable permutation imaginable, the definition of "financial interest" broadly encompasses both compensation arrangements and ownership and investment interests. The Stark Amendments contain a significant number of complicated exceptions and limitations, which variously apply to all financial relationships, compensation arrangements, and ownership and investment interests.

The Stark Amendments operate as a strict liability offense, so a physician doesn't need to be aware of the law or intend to break it for a violation to occur. Violation of the Stark Amendments is punishable by being thrown out of the Medicare program and civil penalties of up to $15,000 plus twice the amount claimed for each service that a person knows (or should have known) should not have been claimed. Although HHS has issued some regulations interpreting the scope of the Stark Amendments, the process has been exceedingly difficult and time-consuming. Enforcement has also been rare.

False Claims

The False Claims Act was a Civil War–era statute, enacted in response to anecdotes of procurement fraud against the Union Army.[10] The original statute included both civil and criminal sanctions, which were subsequently separated into distinct statutory provisions. The FCA creates a cause of action against individuals or entities who knowingly present a false claim to the government. No specific intent to defraud is required; it is sufficient if the defendant acted with "deliberate ignorance" or in "reckless disregard" of the falsity of the statement. Sloppy billing practices, such as failing to review claims carefully before they are submitted, will satisfy this standard. If it can be shown that a representative sample of claims is false, the court will generalize the results to all filed claims. Because of these considerations, an FCA case is much easier to investigate and prosecute than a comparable criminal case.

An FCA claim may be brought by the federal government or private plaintiffs. If a private plaintiff brings the case, the government can elect to take it over or allow the plaintiff to pursue it on his own. Private plaintiffs who sue under the FCA are known as *qui tam* relators and are entitled to a share of the eventual recovery—with the relative share affected by whether the government takes over the case. Historically, the vast majority of the cases that the government does not join have foundered.

The FCA specifies that violators are liable for a statutory penalty of $5,500 to $11,000 per claim, in addition to three times the amount of damages sustained by the government because of the false claim. Because most health care providers typically submit a large number of modest claims, this structure means that statutory penalties generally dwarf actual damages, and quickly rise to staggering levels—as much as $1.1 million for every 100 false claims, irrespective of the dollar value of the false claims. In one case, a provider accused of receiving an overpayment of $245,392 was sued for statutory penalties of $81 million.[11] The stakes in these cases are so large that most defendants are under extreme pressure to settle, and quickly do so. Indeed, virtually all of the precedents involve (generally unsuccessful) motions to dismiss. Thus, the allegations of plaintiffs are almost never tested at trial—a pattern that, I am pleased to report, creates substantial opportunities for mischief on the part of those bringing FCA claims.

These fraud and abuse provisions create a self-reinforcing dynamic that redounds to our benefit. The vast sums of money spent by Medicare create the demand for laws to restrain the avarice of providers. Provider avarice triggers a search for ways around those laws, which, in turn, results in the broadening of those laws. As the laws are broadened, they discourage organizational innovation and market entry and catch more innocent providers. This, in turn, triggers a backlash against the law and widespread violation thereof. Plus, lawyers get rich off each step. What more could we ask for?

the fraud control program works. Although Medicare's fraud control program was well intended, we have, through a variety of skillful measures, successfully redirected it to encourage our larger goals.

First, we ensured that the reach of the fraud statutes would exceed their (functionally defensible) grasp by criminalizing conduct well beyond that which was necessary to protect the program. Indeed, we even criminalized conduct that results in benefits to patients without fiscal harm to the program. That created overwhelming incentives for otherwise law-abiding lawyers and providers to simply ignore the law. Not surprisingly, the same "speakeasy" norms that we observed during Prohibition developed. Professor James Blumstein describes the issue nicely:

> In the current environment it is a truism that the fraud and abuse law is being violated routinely but that those violations are acknowledged as not threatening the public interest. Indeed, they further the public interest and are needed to improve the functioning of the health care marketplace. . . . In sum, the modern American health care industry is akin to a speakeasy—conduct that is illegal is rampant and countenanced by law enforcement officials because the law is so out of sync with the conventional norms and realities of the marketplace and because respected leaders of the industry are performing tasks that, while illegal, are desirable in improving the functioning of the market.[12]

There were predictable consequences when this speakeasy norm came into conflict with the norms of fraud control personnel. For example, in one well-known case, the government charged Columbia/HCA with Medicare fraud, asserting that its use of two sets of cost reports indicated it was intending to break the law—even though most companies in the health care business were reported to use two sets of cost reports.[13] In another high-profile case, the government obtained a settlement of $111 million from National Health Labs, even though the U.S. attorney reportedly conceded that there wasn't a health lawyer in the United States that would have advised his clients against the practices in question.[14] The following sidebar provides details on another notorious case that demonstrates how these anti-fraud statutes serve our larger goals.

Medicare Fraud and Abuse: A Case Study

Consider the case of Dr. Swaran Jain, a psychologist who was convicted under the anti-kickback laws of soliciting and receiving remuneration from a psychiatric hospital for referring patients for admission. The patients actually required hospitalization; the facility was as good as or better than any of the alternatives and provided proper care to each of the patients; and there was no evidence that any patient suffered tangible harm or that the government suffered any adverse fiscal consequences. After a jury convicted Dr. Jain, the court of appeals affirmed the conviction, notwithstanding its observation that "all of the evidence suggests that Dr. Jain intended to provide and did provide his patients with the highest quality psychological services." Yet, he is now a convicted felon for conduct that should be unobjectionable on economic, health policy, and ethical grounds.[15]

The self-referral provisions are subject to similar criticisms, although they compound the problem with their

---

ambitious but highly indeterminate attempt to address any conceivable arrangement between physicians and 10 categories of ancillary services providers. When this indeterminacy is coupled with strict liability, the deleterious consequences of the fraud control regime become even clearer. The self-referral provisions certainly provide little help in differentiating fraudulent and abusive conduct from conduct that is harmless or beneficial to program beneficiaries. Indeed, when the American Health Lawyer's Public Interest Colloquium met to discuss the Medicare fraud and abuse laws, the diverse group of representatives of government, providers, academics, and other involved parties overwhelmingly believed the self-referral provisions were neither effective nor efficient.[16]

Second, we whipped up a frenzy among the public about health care fraud and created the widespread belief that fraud and abuse are pervasive. In fact, no one knows how common fraud and abuse are, but 72 percent of the American public believes that Medicare would have no financial problems if fraud and abuse were eliminated.[17] This perception is utterly uninformed by any connection with reality, but it serves our purposes nonetheless. Over time, Americans will begin to doubt the good faith and reputation for fair dealing that has hitherto prevailed among health care providers. This demoralization will ultimately redound to our benefit—as it has done in other areas.

Finally, the anti-kickback statute helped to embarrass the hospital industry, whose reputation for good deeds (principally providing charity care to those unable to pay) had become a serious problem for us. Hospitals had reasonably interpreted the anti-kickback law as prohibiting them from offering discounts to uninsured and indigent patients because offering selective discounts induces referral—a no-no under this statute. Since hospital "list prices" (which no one ever pays) are staggeringly high, those least able to pay are faced with huge bills, consistent with Medicare regulations requiring reasonable efforts to collect unpaid bills. Various hospitals, both nonprofit and for-profit, then decided to use collection agencies to hound those patients unmercifully. Several hospitals (including Yale–New Haven Hospital) had their debtors arrested as a way of encouraging payment—shades of Dickens!

As if things weren't demonic enough, the lawyers got involved. The Yale Law School students sued Yale–New Haven Hospital on behalf of individuals who had received treatment and were the target of aggressive debt collection for unpaid bills. The Attorney General of Connecticut filed a similar lawsuit. Then, more than 50 health systems across the country were named as defendants in class-action lawsuits led by a well-known plaintiffs' attorney from the tobacco litigation—alleging hospitals had engaged in "price gouging" of the uninsured.[18] Other lawsuits were filed by other lawyers against both not-for-profit and for-profit hospitals, alleging similar concerns. Although many of these lawsuits are objectively frivolous, it's a good day for us anytime we have doctors, lawyers, and hospital administrators at one another's throats.

4. Gluttony

Medicare promotes gluttony among its beneficiaries. At the outset of the Medicare program, the costs of care (both per beneficiary and total) were relatively modest, and beneficiaries were responsible for a substantial percentage of the cost of the care that they received from nonhospital sources. However, the very existence of the Medicare program evoked and encouraged gluttony—and the political consequence of that gluttony was a one-way ratchet that shifted the costs of the Medicare program to the working population and away from Medicare beneficiaries. In essence, we have created a reverse–Robin Hood health care scheme that robs from the poor and working class and gives to the middle class and the rich. This issue has attracted relatively little attention, beyond occasional cutting observations about "single working mothers in Nebraska (often themselves lacking health insurance) footing the bill for gold-plated health care provided to high-income Medicare enrollees in Miami."[1]

This one-way ratchet has operated in all aspects of the Medicare program. As a group, the elderly received far more from the public trough than they ever paid in (and more than is economically sustainable) even before the MMA, which made things substantially worse for younger taxpayers.[2] Due to our hard work, these distributional inequities are not unique to Medicare, but pervade the entire health care marketplace.[3]

The single best confirmation of the gluttony evoked by Medicare was the fate of the Medicare Catastrophic Coverage Act of

1988.[4] Congress passed the Catastrophic Coverage Act with good intentions, overwhelming bipartisan support and the enthusiastic endorsement of groups purporting to represent the elderly, including the American Association of Retired Persons. The Catastrophic Coverage Act created coverage against catastrophic medical expenditures for Medicare beneficiaries. (Coverage against catastrophes is, after all, the core purpose of insurance.) After the legislation precipitated massive opposition among senior citizens, it was repealed less than a year after enactment, in a humiliating about-face for all involved. (Ironically enough, the Catastrophic Coverage Act also provided for prescription drug coverage. Its repeal meant that Congress had to struggle with the problem of prescription drug coverage for senior citizens for another 15 years, until the MMA passed.)

The principal "sin" of the Catastrophic Coverage Act (and I use the term ironically, because the bill was actually exceedingly virtuous and we benefited greatly from its repeal) was that it imposed the costs of expanded coverage on the population that would benefit from the expansion. All senior citizens would have paid a flat $4 monthly premium, with a supplemental premium of 15 percent of one's tax liability imposed on seniors with at least $150 or more of federal income tax. The supplemental premium was capped at $800 for an individual, and $1,600 for a couple. For single seniors with taxable income of $20,000 (or a married couple with taxable income of $30,000), the supplemental premium would have come to $158. The maximum supplemental premium would affect only individuals with taxable income in excess of $45,000 and couples with taxable income in excess of $75,000. According to the Congressional Budget Office, only 36 percent of Medicare recipients would pay any supplemental premium in 1989, while only 5 percent would pay the maximum supplemental premium.

Predictably enough, gluttony turned out to be less appealing when the elderly were presented with the bill, and "open revolt" resulted.[5] Congress was flooded with mail, and there were numerous confrontations with angry constituents when individual representatives returned to their districts. One of the most searing images for a risk-averse representative desirous of reelection was the spectacle of Dan Rostenkowski, House Ways and Means Chairman and one of the most powerful men in Congress, fleeing a crowd of irate senior citizens protesting the Catastrophic Coverage Act. Although Mr. Rostenkowski was reelected, the debacle reinforced the risks of "messing with Medicare" for even the dullest members of Congress. It is for this reason that it became the conventional wisdom in Washington that Medicare was the "third rail of politics"—touch it and you die.[6]

Medicare and the Politics of Protest

On August 17, 1989, Representative Rostenkowski left a meeting in his home district where he had been speaking about the advantages of the Medicare Catastrophic Coverage Act. He was met by a group of 50 senior citizens, who waved signs protesting the fact that they would have to pay more taxes to fund the covered benefit. People shouted "coward," "recall," and "impeach" after Mr. Rostenkowski refused to speak with them and got in his car. One senior citizen (Leona Kozien) even jumped on the hood of Mr. Rostenkowski's car to stop him from leaving—an image beyond even our wildest expectations. After Mr. Rostenkowski got out of the car, he ran a block, where he was picked up

---

by his car and whisked away. The incident resulted in a front-page article in the *Chicago Tribune*, and coverage in the national papers.[7] Mike Royko, a well-known columnist for the *Chicago Tribune*, wrote a piece noting that it wasn't politically smart to have "a little old lady protester winding up on the hood of your car," let alone "jumping out of your car and running away from old people who think they're getting shafted by Congress."[8]

I have reproduced below a photograph from the protest for your viewing pleasure. Ms. Kozien is the woman standing in front of the car, with her hand just above the hood.

MEDICARE BENEFICIARY LEONA KOZIEN MEETS REP. DAN ROSTENKOWSKI'S CAR

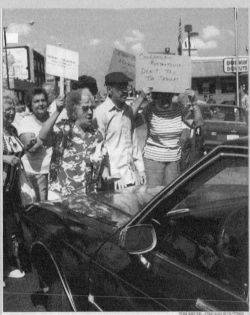

TOM KRUZE—CHICAGO SUN-TIMES
Stunning irony: *Leona Kozien (center front) blocks a car carrying Dan Rostenkowski*

As published in the *Chicago Sun-Times*. Photographer: Tom Cruze. Copyright 1989 by Chicago Sun-Times, Inc. Reprinted with permission.

Everyone involved recognized that opposition was driven by a felicitous (at least from our perspective) combination of gluttony, greed, and selfishness. For example, Senator Lloyd Bentsen noted that "what you have is the wealthier people not wanting to pay an additional premium and wanting it to be more heavily subsidized by the other taxpayers in this country."[9] Senator Robert Packwood stated that the senior citizens who wanted the legislation repealed "all live in Sun City [Arizona] and . . . have incomes of $30,000 or $35,000 or $40,000 a year."[10] In the House, prominent Democrats said the elderly were "ungrateful" and should be left to "stew in their own juices" (Representative Henry Waxman), and that seniors who want long-term care without helping to pay for it should "guess again" (Representative Stark).[11] Representative Stark came closest to the truth about Medicare when he said, "The hell with it."[12] Luckily, no one was listening.

The tone in the media was almost as scathing—the *New York Times* editorialized that "there's little reason to sympathize with the aggrieved affluent elderly" whose complaints were "shortsighted and narrow-minded."[13] In the *New Republic,* one commentator condemned the "selfishness" of the "affluent elderly," and asked, "So long as we continue to provide enormous subsidies to the affluent elderly, why shouldn't they help pay for the poor of their generation?"[14] Television coverage echoed the same themes; on NBC, Andrea Mitchell observed that "the elderly are not against the new benefits—unlimited hospital care, new at-home benefits, prescription drug coverage; they just don't want to pay for them."[15]

Thankfully, the voting power of the elderly has ensured that the "mistake" of the Catastrophic Coverage Act will never be repeated. As the following cartoon exemplifies, every subsequent election cycle has featured increasingly shameless pandering by

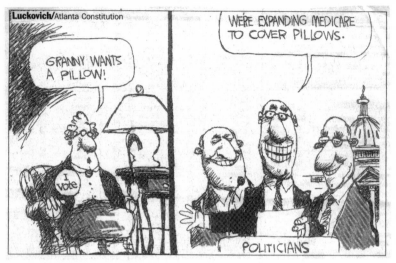

© 1994. By permission of Mike Luckovich and Creators Syndicate, Inc.

both political parties to the preferences of the elderly for more extensive (and more expensive) Medicare coverage.

Fortunately for us, legislators have not limited their pandering to pillows, but have systematically expanded the scope of the program—notwithstanding breathtaking funding shortfalls totaling more than $70 trillion, as described in chapter 10. The most recent and notorious example of this pandering is found in the MMA. Before the MMA, approximately 75 percent of Medicare beneficiaries had prescription drug coverage,[16] with average total drug expenditures of $600 (and out-of-pocket expenditures of $300) per beneficiary.[17] Rather than focus on beneficiaries without prescription drug coverage, or better still on those unable to pay for prescription drugs, Congress enacted the MMA to provide a pharmaceutical benefit for all Medicare beneficiaries that elect to participate.

The design of the benefit reflected even more pandering. To ensure that every senior citizen got some benefit from Part D, the statute provides for reimbursement of 75 percent of the cost of prescription drugs after a deductible of $250. That 75 percent coverage reaches up to $2,250 in total drug expenses. But then to make the benefit "affordable," there is a "donut hole" of zero coverage from $2,250 up to $5,100 of total drug expenses. Above $5,100, Part D pays 95 percent of costs.[18] No rational insurance product looks anything like this, but the politics of pandering is inexorable—as the following illustration exemplifies.

Although competition has eliminated the "donut hole" for many beneficiaries, the MMA is still a testament to the gluttony of Medicare beneficiaries—and that gluttony has dramatically accelerated the day of reckoning that we have worked toward since you first proposed the Medicare program.

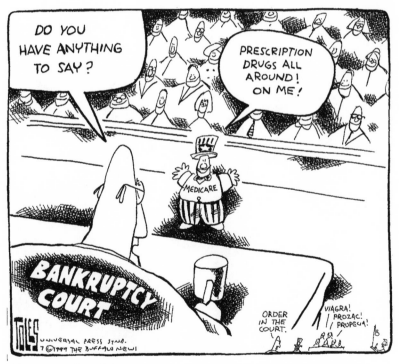

Toles © 1999 *The Buffalo News.* Reprinted with Permission of Universal Press Syndicate. All Rights Reserved.

5. Envy

Envy has been the most disappointing of the seven deadly sins. We have been, at best, only moderately successful at using Medicare to evoke envy among the nonelderly population. Those not covered by Medicare have certainly grown tired of the restrictions and limitations imposed by managed care in the private coverage market. As the last bastion of fee-for-service health care, Medicare is often seen by its enthusiasts as a bonanza of open-ended affordable access to all necessary goods and services without government red tape. Yet, popular envy has been tempered by the realization that Medicare is only "affordable" because of the infusion of hundreds of billions of dollars in subsidies from the rest of the population. There has been no popular uprising in favor of a one-payer system, despite periodic attempts to package it as "Medicare for all."

Part of our problem is that it has proved difficult to persuade people that Medicare is "hassle free"—particularly when providers and prominent members of Congress routinely complain about the inadequacies and inefficiencies of CMS and promise to eliminate it. We can take some credit for this outcome because we persuaded Congress to increase the obligations of CMS while starving them of resources—all the while encouraging Medicare's proponents to brag about its low administrative overhead.[1]

We have had some success in creating envy within the Medicare population by carefully designing the program to maximize hard feelings along geographic lines. Because local costs of production and treatment patterns affect total payments, the cost to the Medicare program (and hence the amount of resources spent per beneficiary) varies greatly among the several states, as well as within those states. Although one state always has to come in last, it is striking how large the variations in payments per beneficiary actually are, even at a statewide level. Payments per beneficiary range from $3,053 in Iowa (51st) to $10,373 in the District of Columbia.[2] Of course, these figures are complicated by the fact that people can travel from one state to another to receive medical care—meaning that the Medicare program's spending on their care is not credited to their state (the numerator), even though they are counted in the denominator. Of course, the opposite applies to people who travel to a state to receive health care—the cost of their care is counted in the numerator, but they are not counted in the denominator.[3]

After one controls for that problem, there are still significant geographic variations in treatment costs. Indeed, these payment disparities are so large that one group of commentators has estimated that we could buy every Medicare beneficiary in Florida who agreed to receive their health care in Minnesota a fully loaded Lexus and the Medicare program would still come out ahead.[4] Scholars at Dartmouth Medical School helped surface some of these payment disparities, but Medicare Part C helped draw attention to the issue as well.[5]

To administer Medicare Part C, CMS must determine and publish the average cost of treating Medicare beneficiaries on a county-by-county basis. CMS uses these figures to determine how much it should pay for the care provided to Medicare beneficiaries enrolled in Part C.[6] Because the cost of treatment varies so much throughout the United States, the resulting amounts are enough to pay for "gold-plated" benefits in some counties, and only "bare-bones" coverage in other counties.[7] Once again, these payment and coverage disparities have helped trigger modest amounts of envy among Medicare beneficiaries.

Geographically based envy has also precipitated a "formula fight" among the states, complete with litigation,[8] coalitions of aggrieved states and senior citizens,[9] coverage in newspapers and editorials,[10] and statements from concerned legislators.[11] As the following advertisement reflects, certain state medical societies have been particularly insistent that their states are being short-changed by the Medicare program.[12] These interest groups have had great success in persuading their elected representatives to change Medicare's reimbursement formulas, so the Medicare money train unloads their "fair share."

We have also had considerable success with creating envy across types of providers. Those currently included within Medicare compare their payment rate with that of other covered providers and ceaselessly agitate to have "their" services compensated more highly. Providers who are excluded from Medicare agitate to be included. Medical device manufacturers lobby to have their devices covered and lobby against Medicare's attempts to impose a cost-effectiveness test on coverage.[13]

Interestingly, pharmaceutical manufacturers are the only organized group that has shown no real interest in expanding their presence in Medicare. Indeed, they lobbied heavily against adding an outpatient prescription drug benefit—until it became clear there was going to be a Medicare Part D. At that point they switched course and focused on minimizing the government's ability to exercise its newly created purchasing power—and quite predictably got hammered for doing so.

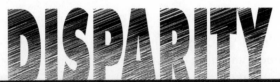

If Americans pay the same Medicare taxes, why is there such a huge disparity in Medicare reimbursement?

GEM Member Organizations as of September 2002

American Academy of Family Physicians

Idaho Medical Association

Iowa Medical Society

Kansas Medical Society

Maine Medical Association

Medical Association of the State of Alabama

Minnesota Medical Association

Montana Medical Association

Nebraska Medical Association

New Hampshire Medical Society

New Mexico Medical Society

North Dakota Medical Association

Oklahoma State Medical Association

Oregon Medical Association

South Dakota Medical Association

Utah Medical Association

Vermont Medical Society

Wisconsin Medical Society

Did you know that for a left heart catheterization, physicians in San Francisco are reimbursed $2,161.03 but physicians in Nebraska are reimbursed just $1,349.07 (a 38% decrease)? If you have the same procedure in Puerto Rico, physicians receive just $1,107.00 (a 48% decrease). Did you know that a mid-level office visit is reimbursed at $63.07 in San Francisco and just $45.05 (a 29% decrease) in South Dakota?

Geographic Equity in Medicare (GEM) Coalition

Americans everywhere pay equal premiums to support Medicare, yet there is substantial geographic disparity in patient services and physician reimbursement levels in the Medicare Part B program. The degree of this disparity is unjustified and inherently unfair — and is having an increasingly negative impact on patient care and access in many parts of the United States.

GEM is formed to remedy this alarming inequity. The member organizations believe that federal policymakers must assign a high priority to eliminating Geographic Practice Cost Indices and other components of the Medicare Part B program that result in this inappropriate and inequitable reimbursement to the tens of thousands of physicians across this country providing medical care to millions of Medicare beneficiaries. The critical nature of this problem compels immediate attention and action. For over a decade members of this coalition and others working through the Geographic Coalition have addressed these gross disparities. Productive improvements in Medicare Plus Choice helped lay the foundation to continue to address these inequities experienced by many patients and their physicians.

We call on members of the United States Senate to support legislation that will restore fairness to Medicare Part B reimbursement, such as the Improving Our Well-Being Act (S.2873) sponsored by Iowa Senator Charles Grassley.

6. Sloth

Medicare fosters sloth in two important groups: legislators and program administrators. To be sure, Congress tinkers with numerous aspects of Medicare on a more or less annual basis, but it has paid almost no attention to the long-term financial problems facing Medicare. As outlined previously, Medicare's financing is a ticking time bomb that will explode within the next two generations. The sooner this problem is addressed, the less severe the resulting dislocations will be. Yet, legislative sloth ensures that any solution will be deferred until a true crisis emerges—and by the time the crisis emerges, legislators will have more difficulty solving the problem. (So much for the oft-heard claims about the superior ability of government to mind the interests of future generations and attend to long-term problems. Due to your diligent efforts, this particular fairy tale has become widely accepted in certain political circles in the United States. Yet, neither theory nor practice provides any basis for believing that the political system will effectively protect the interests of future voters—let alone future nonvoters.)

Program administrators are also affected by sloth, at least with regard to quality and, to a lesser extent, fraud control. When one is purchasing health care, cost, quality, and access are all important. Yet, Medicare program administrators care a lot about cost, less about access, and, at least historically, not at all about quality.[1] This sloth is no accident. Indeed, at your behest, Medicare's fundamental structure was designed at every turn to focus program administrators on cost and access and to discount quality.[2] As noted in chapter 2, the Medicare statute explicitly specifies that any provider who meets the entry requirements is entitled to participate in the program, and that patients are free to choose any provider who will have them. Thus, CMS has very little ability to exclude providers who deliver poor quality care, or to reward providers whose quality is exemplary. Indeed, CMS's minimal efforts to steer patients by designating "centers of excellence" for cardiac and orthopedic surgery triggered extensive discontent among providers, who feared losing patients and revenues.[3]

Similarly, the administrative structure of Medicare also helped contribute to administrative sloth. Because all bills are processed by carriers and intermediaries, CMS has little responsibility for the day-to-day administration of the program. Those carriers and intermediaries view their job as paying bills as quickly and cheaply as possible, which CMS wants as well.[4] The result is to encourage sloth even in those instances when CMS would otherwise be inclined to act aggressively.

It was also an act of demonic genius to draw the original administrators of Medicare from the ranks of the Social Security Administration. SSA administrators had considerable experience and expertise in running a program that was based on the payment of specified amounts to qualifying beneficiaries and no experience whatsoever with purchasing health care services. The predictable result was that program administrators were extremely focused on (1) whether beneficiaries had access to the statutorily specified services, (2) the total amount of money required to accomplish that objective, and (3) the prompt and efficient processing and payment of claims. Program administrators paid relatively little attention to everything else. Shoveling money out the door to purchase health care services for qualifying beneficiaries is, of course, not the same thing as purchasing high-quality health care.

These patterns have continued to the present day. Even if program administrators were inclined to exercise their purchasing power on behalf of program beneficiaries, the basic structure of Medicare—the requirements for public notice and comment on virtually everything it does, the chronic underfunding of administrative capacity, and the multiplicity of tasks that CMS is charged with—means that sloth will continue to prevail, regardless of the enthusiasm, hard work, and promises made by program administrators.

Finally, in a diabolical stroke of genius, you have succeeded in undermining all attempts to rouse administrators from their sloth through the judicious use of political oversight. Any attempt by CMS to transform itself from a passive payer of bills to an active manager with broad responsibility for beneficiary health—using selective contracting and payment for performance, among other tools—will necessarily result in shifts in patient flows (and payments) among providers. Adversely affected providers lobby heavily to forestall this fate. The outcome of such disputes is determined by the political power of those involved, instead of the quality and efficiency with which they deliver health care services.[5] Thus, political oversight ends up either shutting down CMS initiatives or hijacking them to serve the self-interest of providers.

Small-scale demonstration projects have triggered similar dynamics: when a demonstration project is successful, CMS lacks the authority to implement it more broadly, and when a demonstration is unsuccessful, political constraints can make it impossible to terminate.[6] Political opposition killed at least one such demonstration project before it even got off the ground.[7] Those advocating such efforts will also be legislatively savaged for their troubles. As such, sloth has predictably become the dominant strategy for risk-averse program administrators and legislators.

7. Lust

The Medicare program induces lust for program expansion and political power, chiefly among members of the Democratic Party. Democrats lust to extend the "security" of Medicare to the balance of the population and ceaselessly campaign to do so. These unknowing pawns write endlessly about the supposed virtues of a government-run health system, monopolizing the op-ed pages of major newspapers and medical journals. In a real tribute to your powers, these advocates actually believe they are engaged in *God's* work! Although we occasionally encourage their efforts by allowing public referendums on the adoption of a one-payer system and periodically tantalize them with proposals to add the "near elderly" to Medicare, we adhere to your original plan to resist making Medicare universal until we have completely bankrupted the United States. As the cartoon below indicates, inviting more people aboard a sinking ship only makes it sink faster—and if it sinks too fast, Americans might wake up and smell the coffee.

Medicare and Sex

No cheap shots about Medicare and Viagra here. No, sir. We draw the line at that kind of easy laugh. Well, maybe just one. Did you hear the one about the guy who joined a Medicare HMO because he thought it covered his Viagra? It didn't.[1]

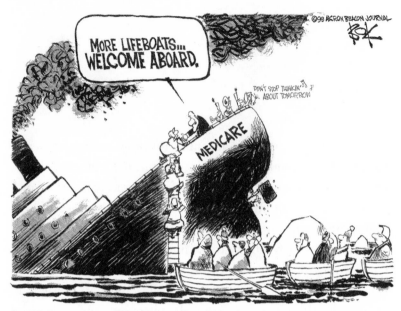

© 1998. By permission of Chip Bok and Creators Syndicate, Inc.

Stated more formally, allowing everyone into Medicare makes the program impossible to sustain in its current form because the subsidies that sustain Medicare are achievable only if there are sufficient chumps *outside* the program to pay the necessary funds *into* the program. Of course, "Medicare for all" would be sustainable if global budgets were used to control program expenditures—but that approach will necessitate substantial rationing—and there is no enthusiasm for that policy strategy, even among those who would otherwise accept our "spin" at face value.

Program beneficiaries understand this problem perfectly well. The demise of the Clinton plan was inevitable once it became clear that the plan would "take" from the elderly and "give" to the uninsured.[2] We are far better off delaying the day of reckoning by a few years and allowing the gluttony of Medicare beneficiaries and the passage of time to increase the number of unsustainable commitments—meaning that the American Republic's fall from grace will be even more precipitous.

Medicare also provides Democrats with the tools to satisfy their lust for power. Of course, the lust for power is innate in all politicians and political parties. However, Democrats disproportionately emphasize Medicare in their appeals to the electorate, which is consistent with their basic position that the "highest purpose of government is to send people checks in the mail."[3] The proof of these claims is in the pudding. Political polling has consistently demonstrated that voters trust the Democrats more than the Republicans when it comes to Medicare.[4] Exploiting this asymmetry, Democrats use Medicare as a bludgeon against their Republican adversaries at every conceivable turn regardless of the actual differences between the parties, the bipartisanship of the effort, and the financial straits in which Medicare finds itself.

For example, in the 2002 congressional election, one Maryland Democratic candidate argued that his Republican opponent was "anti-Medicare" because she voted in 1988 for the Catastrophic Coverage Act—along with the rest of the Maryland congressional delegation (most of whom are Democrats) and an overwhelming majority of Congress.[5] More generally, the Democratic Party's "talking points" for the 2002 election reduced to the claim that Republicans did not care about the elderly, a fact "demonstrated" by their refusal to enact a Medicare prescription drug benefit even though the (Republican) House had actually passed a Medicare prescription drug benefit—albeit one not to the taste of the Democrats. In the 2000 presidential election, Vice President Gore repeatedly accused the Republicans of planning to cut Medicare to pay for tax cuts.[6] In the 1992 and 1996 presidential elections, President Clinton was particularly effective at using Medicare to score political points against the Republicans, even using it to recover from the devastating losses suffered by the Democrats in the 1994 election.[7] Indeed, the basis for President Clinton's 1996 reelection campaign was referred to by party operatives as M^2E^2, or Me-Me, short for Medicare, Medicaid, Education, and the Environment.[8]

These efforts have been extraordinarily successful. Significant portions of the elderly population distrust Republicans when it comes to Medicare—even though the financial differences between the Republican and Democratic proposals for Medicare are generally exceedingly modest in percentage terms (if not in raw dollars).[9] The Democratic message has been quite effective in overcoming the collective action problems of organizing the elderly, but it has been less successful in creating broad-based confidence in the program. In a recent poll, approximately half of the young women polled thought that the soap opera *General Hospital* would outlast Medicare.[10]

Chris Matthews offers a larger philosophical perspective on these issues. Matthews divides:

> the parties into the "mommy party," the Democrats, and the "daddy party," the Republicans. When times are good, you turn to mom, who promises to provide more services and more compassion, and demands less personal responsibility. But when threats loom, Americans turn to dad, who takes no guff from us but also reaches for the Winchester hanging over the front door when hostile strangers approach.[11]

As the quintessential mommy-party program, Medicare has been a critical part of the platform for Democrats and the key to victory in many swing districts. I note in passing that it was only with considerable last-minute lobbying that we were able to forestall attempts to rename HCFA the Medicare and Medicaid

Agency (MaMA). We were greatly aided in our lobbying efforts by the ideological implications of the name change. HHS Secretary Thompson conceded that he had been considering the agency MaMA, but noted that "women found that acronym insulting. Also, it reinforced an image of the agency as paternalistic, or in this case maternalistic, at a time when President Bush wants Medicare beneficiaries to take more responsibility for their health insurance options."[12] Had HCFA been renamed the Medicare and Medicaid Agency, we would have had MaMA running Medicare—allowing even the dimmest to see the implications of your plans.

Finally, I am happy to report the dynamic described in this chapter is not unique to the United States, but prevails everywhere we have introduced Medicare-type programs. Thus, in Canada, for Liberals, "medicare is an ideological achievement, a propaganda device and an election issue."[13] In Britain, Labour routinely blasts the Conservatives over the National Health Service. It is a tribute to your demonic genius that we can use Medicare to further our mission on a wholesale basis, instead of continuing to buy souls at retail.

8. Anger

Medicare triggers anger mostly among members of the Republican Party. As previously noted, the Democrats have been quite successful at positioning themselves as the protectors of the Medicare program and of program beneficiaries. The Republicans cannot "outbid" the Democrats on Medicare, as there is no limit to the amounts the Democrats are willing to spend on the program. In addition, Democrats have routinely and effectively demagogued Republican efforts to make even minor revisions to the financing of Medicare and its delivery options.[1]

Not surprisingly, Republicans are angry about the effectiveness with which a large command-and-control program, which is inexorably gobbling up an ever-increasing share of federal tax revenues, has become a seemingly sacrosanct feature of American politics. Their anger is magnified because Medicare was quite unpopular among the conservative wing of the Republican Party to begin with. The madder they get, the less credible their efforts to escape the box in which Your Eminence has placed them.

Interestingly, there is some indication that the passage of the MMA caused the parties to adopt each other's deadly sins. When Congress was considering the Republican-sponsored bill that ultimately became Part D, anger became the dominant Democratic response. Senator Edward Kennedy's over-the-top rhetoric makes the point clear: "Who do you trust? The HMO-coddling, drug-company loving, Medicare-destroying, Social-Security-hating Bush administration? Or do you trust Democrats, who created

Medicare and will fight with you to defend it every day of every week of every year?"[2] House Democratic Leader Nancy Pelosi warned a rally that "Democrats will work day and night against this shameful Republican bill . . . this Republican hoax leaves most seniors and the disabled worse off than before. . . . Republicans have been clear—they want to kill Medicare."[3] When the bill passed the House after an extended period for voting, Representative Pelosi issued a statement that excoriated the Republicans for "stealing" the vote "by hook or crook" and claimed that "Republicans [were] not fit to be in the majority in this House" and their action "brought dishonor to this institution."[4]

The rhetorical low point however, came during the debate over the MMA, when Representative Ed Markey warned:

> Watch out, grandma. Watch out, grandpa. The GOP is selling snake oil off the back of a wagon, and, boy, do they have a prescription for you, further weakening the foundation of Medicare for the seniors who need it most. This is a black day for Medicare. You know, GOP used to stand for Grand Old Party. Now it stands for get old people.[5]

Of course, from our perspective, this new rhetorical low was a welcome development, as it was a new high-water mark for Democratic anger over Medicare. Although Democrats have not completely abandoned lust, their dominant deadly sin has since become anger.

Republicans, on the other hand, allowed their lust for political power to overwhelm their principles. As an article in the *New England Journal of Medicine* noted, Republicans were "determined to break the long hold that Democrats have maintained on Medicare as a political asset."[6] Doing so required them to throw more money at a program that was already in serious financial difficulty, and that they disliked on ideological grounds independent of its financial straits. Provisions added to appeal to Senate Democrats made the vote even less appealing for many Republicans. As Speaker Dennis Hastert acknowledged, "A lot of our folks, the hard-right guys, are not for Medicare. It's an entitlement they don't want to add on to."[7] The net result is that some conservative Republicans became even angrier about Medicare, because other Republicans were so lustful for power that they voted to expand an out-of-control entitlement.

More broadly, whether motivated by lust or anger, Medicare has become an equal-opportunity club for use against one's political opponents, regardless of party affiliation. As a former Democratic representative ruefully observed:

> There is no better subject for effective negative campaigning than a vote to slow the growth of the Medicare program with whatever cost-cutting or benefit-denying or premium-increasing it may involve. Any member knows that however good or decent a Medicare reform bill may be, his opponent in his next campaign will use a vote for that bill against him. It does not take a clairvoyant to see what the television commercial will be: "When he had the chance to protect Medicare, the program that provides health care to all of us in our vulnerable old age, our congressman, [your name here], voted instead to protect the special interests by increasing the premiums." Forget about all the cuts in payment to doctors and hospitals, which pay for 90 percent of the funding changes. "He voted to protect the special interests by increasing the premiums we all must pay for doctor and hospital care." An opponent has to be an idiot not to make campaign hay with that vote.[8]

Thus, Medicare has become a cost-effective scourge of both political parties, allowing each party to satisfy its lust for power and express its anger, while undermining each party's ability to govern effectively once in office.

In short, we have achieved the best of both worlds, with anger and lust no longer the exclusive province of one party or the other. Instead, there is bipartisan sharing of the sins—and what could be better for us than that? The resulting poisoning of legislative politics, whether it results from the combination of Democratic lust and Republican anger, or Republican lust and Democratic anger, ensures that any reforms to Medicare will not address its fundamental structural flaws. As such, the program remains on autopilot, rather like the *Titanic* bearing down on an iceberg. Of course, the sinking of the *Titanic* closed relatively few of our open accounts. The temptations of Medicare, its impending implosion, and the resulting demoralization will add tens of millions to our ranks.

9. Vanity

I close with your favorite sin, vanity. To some extent, this sin affects virtually everyone touched by Medicare, but the group whose vanity is most greatly affected is health policy analysts. (Of course, congressional vanity comes in second. But on the subject of congressional vanity, like the sun rising in the east, what more can be said?) Almost without exception, health policy analysts have hailed the virtues of Medicare and excused its dysfunctions, reasoning *sub silentio* that a program offering a rotten benefit package and mediocre health care is better than no program at all. Of course, it is no accident that virtually every one of these health policy analysts is an enthusiastic member of the Democratic Party, for whom the 1960s remains the best of times. Among this group, we actually get a two-for-one effect, as lust and vanity work together in a synergistic fashion.

This vanity takes several distinct forms. One form of vanity is the refusal of health policy analysts to acknowledge the highly variable quality of care provided to Medicare beneficiaries. Normally, policy analysts are stereotypical "goo-goos." As you know, a "goo-goo" is a "good-government" type. They can be counted on to write long, dull, scolding editorials in major newspapers, bemoaning both the latest excesses of the free market and government waste, and advocating for more and better regulatory oversight of whatever offends them. Goo-goos normally insist on the dotting of every *i* and the crossing of every *t* before allowing government money to be spent on anything. Yet, in Medicare, the same analysts have bestowed their blessing on a program that systematically and routinely pays (and frequently overpays!) for the mistreatment of the vulnerable Americans who depend on Medicare. Ironically, these are the same vulnerable Americans for whom goo-goos' hearts generally bleed.

The second form of vanity is the failure of health policy analysts to appreciate the "sauce for the goose" implications of the precedents they have created around the use of Medicare's purchasing power. In most hospitals, Medicare is the single largest purchaser of health care services. As such, health policy analysts (consistent with their goo-goo inclinations) have eagerly tied the acceptance of Medicare money to a variety of our schemes. These schemes impose ancillary restraints on hospitals that undermine their continued viability, condition payment on the satisfaction of every jot and tittle of the thousands of pages of rules and regulations surrounding Medicare (the drafting, interpretation, and enforcement of which provide steady employment to the lawyers who have sold their souls to us in exchange for professional success), or simply impose substantial administrative burdens for no good result.

Fortunately (at least from our perspective), the health policy community never realized that these precedents could be turned on their favorite causes, as the spending power can be used to bat from both sides of the political plate. Indeed, federal funding can be used to require private parties to implement activities that are anathema to health policy analysts, their patrons, and their supporters. Conversely, federal funding can be used to require private parties to terminate activities that are near and dear to the hearts of the same health policy analysts, their patrons, and their supporters. For example, the Solomon Amendments can be used to force universities and law schools to grant equal access to the military for recruiting purposes. The False Claims Act, which requires regulatory compliance with all federal laws, can be used against institutions whose affirmative action programs do not comply with strict constitutional requirements—and the billions of dollars at stake in Medicare will encourage these institutions to settle on almost any terms. Any harebrained idea that occurs to some junior staffer in Congress or midlevel bureaucrat in HHS can be packaged and deployed as an explicit exercise of the spending power. Of course, each change in administration will bring about a dramatic shift in the substantive obligations imposed on all recipients of federal funds. Over time, all recipients will be forced to implement some activities inconsistent with their self-framed missions. This campaign will further our larger agenda of spreading misery and despair.

The third manifestation of the vanity of health policy analysts is their enthusiasm for what I will charitably describe as "asymmetric arguments." When the Medicare "trust fund" is "flush," analysts rebut critics of the program with the observation that Medicare is on sound fiscal footing. When the projected insolvency date grows closer, the same analysts rebut critics by claiming that the "trust fund" is a meaningless accounting convention and financial projections are inherently unreliable.

Another example of this preference for asymmetric arguments involves the "case" that was made for expanding Medicare to include prescription drug coverage. Many health policy analysts juxtaposed the presence of prescription drug coverage in the private employment–based coverage market with its absence in Medicare and assumed they had made the case for program modification. Yet, when it is pointed out that the private coverage market has embraced an array of supply- and demand-side restrictions on access to care, and that it might be prudent to reform

Medicare in an analogous fashion to control program costs, health policy analysts routinely responded that changes in the private market need not be reflected in Medicare. No explanation is offered for why taxpayers should subsidize a system for the elderly that has coverage features that are more generous than those the taxpayers are willing and able to buy for themselves. "Sauce for the goose," anyone?

The fourth form of vanity is the insistence of many health policy analysts that compulsory government-mandated charity (i.e., Medicare) is so important as a symbol of solidarity that Americans should continue and expand the program—regardless of the distributional consequences, mediocre quality, and dire financial projections—simply because at one point in time, one Congress and one president thought it was a good idea. P. J. O'Rourke concisely explained the moral vanity associated with such a stance:

> There is no virtue in compulsory government charity, and there is no virtue in advocating it. A politician who portrays himself as "caring" and "sensitive" because he wants to expand the government's charitable programs is merely saying that he's willing to try to do good with other people's money. Well, who isn't? And a voter who takes pride in supporting such programs is telling us that he'll do good with his own money—if a gun is held to his head.[1]

Of course, we depend heavily on the moral vanity of health policy analysts, and their continued willingness to guzzle communitarian Kool-Aid, to maintain our Medicare brand on "the side of the angels." Best of all, we didn't even have to offer them anything to endorse our product—they actually believe in it! You just can't buy that kind of loyalty.

The final form of vanity is the inability of health policy analysts to perceive the importance of exit and exit rights. In a well-functioning market, vendors decide whether to deal or not. Refusal to deal sends a useful signal about the terms that are being offered. Indeed, exit is a critical component of well-functioning markets, as it ensures that resources are diverted from lower- to higher-valued uses. Yet, in Medicare, health policy analysts treat exit as a mark of disloyalty (as when Medicare managed care organizations decide to pull out of Part C) or as an overt attempt to subvert the self-evident virtues of the program (as when physicians decline to accept new Medicare patients or try to contract with them privately). The criticisms leveled at physicians offering "concierge care" reflect a similar lack of understanding of the importance of exit rights (as well as of basic economics).

Admittedly, it is unclear whether the opposition of health policy analysts to exit rights is attributable to their complete ignorance of economics, their position as academics (who developed tenure to constrain the exercise of exit rights), or both. It is difficult to determine which effect dominates because most health policy analysts are academics and most academics are ignorant of economics.

Regardless of where one comes out on this issue, vanity clearly plays a role in the willingness of health policy analysts to hail Medicare's "virtues," whitewash its faults, and attack those who do not share their faith in the Medicare program. Perhaps the best explanation of this behavior was offered by Saul Bellow: "A great deal of intelligence can be invested in ignorance when the need for illusion is deep."[2]

10. Undermining American Virtues

As you presciently recognized in your memo proposing Medicare, a program incorporating the seven deadly sins would never attain its intended objectives unless we also undermined the American virtues that would otherwise impede our plans. The two distinctively American virtues that most directly threatened our plans were thrift and truthfulness. These virtues figured prominently in the lives of the Founders. Benjamin Franklin celebrated the importance of thrift in numerous influential writings, and George Washington was renowned as the politician who could not tell a lie. American politicians routinely celebrate these virtues, even if they do not invariably display them. The near universality of these virtues in the American population made it much more difficult for our plans to proceed on schedule. Thus, we attacked these virtues using entitlement programs, with Medicare acting as the central tine in our pitchfork.

Thrift

As you know, Medicare's financing provides that revenues secured from current taxpayers fund the medical expenses of current beneficiaries—frequently referred to as "pay-as-you-go" financing. Everyone knows that Medicare spending is increasing dramatically, in both relative and absolute terms. Demographic projections and the ever-increasing cost of health care ensure that the program's economics are simply unsustainable. The basic problem was nicely framed by a former undersecretary of the Treasury in a 2002 speech:

Think of the federal government as a gigantic insurance company (with a side line business in national defense and homeland security) which only does its accounting on a cash basis—only counting premiums and payouts as they go in and out the door. An insurance company with cash accounting is not really an insurance company at all. It is an accident waiting to happen.

This particular insurance company, it turns out, has made promises to its policy holders that have a current value of $20 trillion or so (give or take a few trillion) in excess of the current value of the revenues that it expects to receive. A real insurance company could try to grow its way out by raising its premiums and its earnings on investments faster than its liabilities. The federal government, however, would have to raise taxes or borrow faster than it increases outlays.[1]

This is not an idiosyncratic perspective of an isolated government official. Medicare has a board of trustees that is required by law to report annually on the fiscal health of the program. These reports provide a first-rate barometer of our success. As the summary of the most recent report from the trustees stated,

> The fundamentals of the financial status of Social Security and Medicare remain problematic under the intermediate economic and demographic assumptions. . . . Expenditures of Medicare's Hospital Insurance (HI) Trust Fund that pays hospital benefits are projected to exceed taxes and other dedicated revenues in 2006, with annual cash flow deficits expected to continue and to grow rapidly after 2010 as baby boomers begin to retire. The projected growing deficits in both programs will exhaust HI trust fund reserves in 2018 and Social Security reserves in 2040, under current financing arrangements. In addition, the Medicare Supplementary Medical Insurance (SMI)

Trust Fund that pays for physician services and the new prescription drug benefit will require substantial increases over time in both general revenue financing and beneficiary premium charges. . .We do not believe the currently projected long-run growth rates of Social Security or Medicare are sustainable under current financing arrangements.[2]

Although this statement is from the 2006 trustees' report, there is no material difference between it and the trustees' report from almost any year since Medicare began, other than changes in some of the dates. The most striking thing about these observations is that they are now so routine they are widely ignored—a point emphasized by the following cartoon. We are literally hiding your

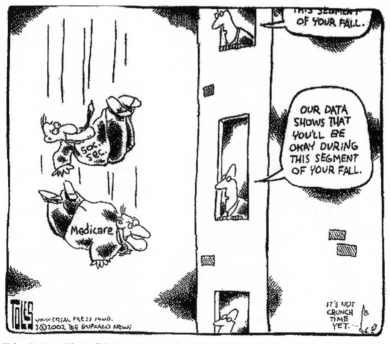

Toles © 2002 *The Buffalo News.* Reprinted with Permission of Universal Press Syndicate. All Rights Reserved.

plan in plain view! Remarkably enough, in a country whose Founders prided themselves on thrift, we have succeeded in "defining deviancy down" to the point that only the imminent "bankruptcy" of the Part A "trust fund" (i.e., less than seven years) will attract any legislative attention whatsoever.[3] (Not at all coincidentally, the number of years is the same as the number of deadly sins). Thus, only the equivalent of "being hanged in a fortnight" will rouse the political process from its sloth—and as noted previously, the consistent approach when attempting "reform" is to fix the short term and ignore the (far more problematic) long term.[4]

To be sure, Medicare's short-term financial prospects are about the same as they have always been—tenuous at best and never once exceeding 28 years to exhaustion of the "trust fund." Indeed, this figure makes it clear that the Part A "trust fund" has not been on an actuarially sound footing (i.e., that which would be expected of a private annuity) at any time since its creation.

The extent of our success in obliterating thrift among the American public becomes crystal clear if one examines the debates over the MMA. Even without a prescription drug benefit, Medicare was projected to suck up a substantial percentage of federal tax revenues. Adding new benefits only worsened the structural deficit of the Medicare program. Consider Figure 10-1, which was available to Congress before it enacted the MMA. The figure projects spending on Medicare as a share of the total federal budget without a prescription drug benefit and then with the Republican and Democratic proposals for a prescription drug benefit. It is clear from this chart that even without a prescription drug benefit, Medicare spending was going to crowd out most other government expenditures. Yet, Congress still enacted the MMA, despite these clear warnings.

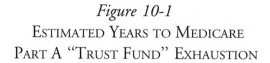

Figure 10-1
ESTIMATED YEARS TO MEDICARE
PART A "TRUST FUND" EXHAUSTION

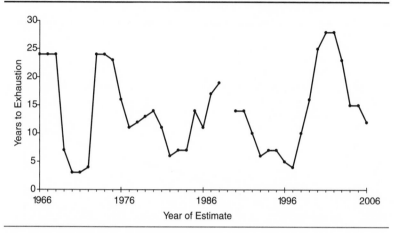

SOURCE: Annual Reports of the Board of Trustees of the Federal Hospital Insurance Trust Fund, 1966–1999.

The extent to which Medicare—with its "promise now, pay later" approach—has succeeded in undermining the distinctively American virtue of thrift becomes frighteningly clear when one computes the present value of the Medicare program's future financial shortfalls. Without even counting the prescription drug benefit, Congress would have to deposit $54.6 trillion in an interest-bearing savings account to cover Medicare's future financial shortfalls. Throw in an additional $16.2 trillion for the prescription drug benefit. Together, that is $70.8 trillion— roughly five times the annual gross domestic product of the United States. If one simply focuses on the next 75 years and only on Part A, the figure is smaller—$11.3 trillion.[5] But the necessary remedies for even this dramatically smaller figure are still drastic: an immediate and permanent 121-percent increase

77

Figure 10-2
PERCENT OF FEDERAL INCOME TAX
DEVOTED TO MEDICARE WITH AND
WITHOUT DRUG BENEFIT (2003 EST.)

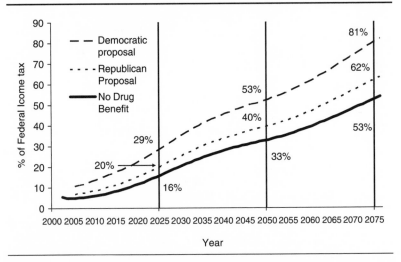

SOURCE: Calculations by Andrew Rettenmaier, Private Enterprise Research Center, Texas A&M University, based on 2002 Medicare Trustees Report, CBO Testimony, March 22, 2001, and March 7, 2002.

in the tax on wages that finance Part A or an immediate and permanent 51-percent reduction in Part A benefits.[6] If these actions are delayed, the remedies will have to be even more drastic.

Of course, given the political dynamics of Medicare, neither of these eventualities will occur. Instead, as the MMA reflects, all the pressures are to expand the program and find money to fund it—not to bring its spending under control.

To summarize, we are lucky that no one has (so far) "connected the dots" of the following fundamental features of Medicare:

- Incessant focus on short-term viability,
- Unsustainable long-term promises,
- Each generation pays for those that preceded it,
- Continuous addition of new participants to finance past promises, and
- Continued participation ensured with appeals to security/fidelity/solidarity.

If these dots are ever connected, people will realize that Medicare is a pyramid scheme structured on an intergenerational basis. All of our nongovernment pyramid schemes have been shut down by the authorities as soon as they are discovered, on the grounds that those who were suckered at the outset have no right to share their misery with others. The legal system imposes harsh penalties on pyramid scheme organizers, because defrauding hundreds or thousands of people is much worse than defrauding a handful of people. Indeed, if anyone other than the United States government were running the Medicare program, those responsible would already be serving long prison terms for fraud.

In like fashion, those responsible for the original Medicare cost estimates would face serious jail time if the federal securities laws applied to their efforts. As the following figure reflects, the only year in which the original estimates for Part A were even close to actual expenditures was the first year of the program—a fact that helps explain why the Johnson administration started looking for solutions to what they believed to be "out-of-control" spending within a year of Medicare getting under way. Finally, if the federal securities laws applied, many members of the executive and legislative branches would be liable for their ceaseless misrepresentations about Medicare's long-term ability to continue providing coverage to program beneficiaries.

Figure 10-3
MEDICARE HOSPITAL SPENDING:
1965 PROJECTIONS VS. ACTUAL

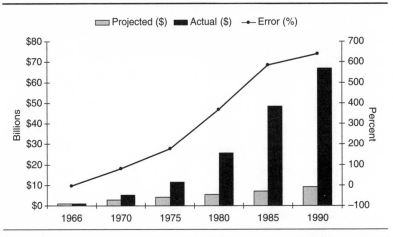

SOURCE: Richard Epstein, *Mortal Peril: Our Inalienable Right to Health Care?* (Reading, Massachusetts: Addison-Wesley, 1997), p. 149.

Given these risks, it was prudent of you to position Medicare as a sacred intergenerational trust. The result of this framing is that all the political pressures are to preserve, if not expand, the pyramid scheme.

Despite our repeated efforts to disguise the truth about Medicare through the endless repetition of misleading rhetoric (principally the terms "trust fund" and "lockbox") many Americans are coming to realize that Medicare is, in fact, little more than a thinly disguised intergenerational pyramid scheme. Indeed, no less a "New Democratic" authority than the *New Republic* has been forced to observe, "If there's a big problem with Medicare these days, it's the program's lack of long-term financial viability."[7] Thankfully, our framing of the Medicare program as a

---

Medicare and Enron

As noted previously, the present value of Medicare's unfunded liabilities are $70.8 trillion. At the time of its bankruptcy filing, Enron claimed liabilities of $27 billion and assets of $61 billion. Even if one assumes that Enron had no assets whatsoever, its liabilities are less than 0.04 percent of Medicare's unfunded liabilities. Yet, the *New Republic* has been the scourge of all those associated with Enron (no matter how distantly), even as it suggests that we should reconfigure the nation's health care along the lines of Medicare. Go figure.

---

sacred intergenerational trust has significantly dampened the outrage that would otherwise result; the *New Republic* would not have been nearly as complacent had the sentence been "if there's a big problem with Enron these days, it's the company's lack of long-term financial viability." Of course, the principal difference between Medicare and Enron is that Medicare's "lack of long-term financial viability" is much worse than Enron's.

Although we have largely stifled the criticisms that pyramid schemes usually engender, we must expect the Medicare program (and its financing) to come under increased scrutiny in the coming years. We have already contacted our lobbyists on K Street and at various think tanks, who stand ready to defend the "virtue" of the Medicare program from its all-too-correct critics. The good news is that our efforts at destroying public education in the United States (along with our systematic resistance to vouchers)

have rendered a large chunk of the population functionally innu-
merate. The impassioned defenses of Medicare offered by most
health policy analysts will accordingly be resolved at the level
of emotional rhetoric, instead of through simple addition and
subtraction.

Truthfulness

As you predicted, entitlement programs have provided numerous opportunities for political dissembling. The ceaseless use of
misleading terminology (e.g., "trust fund" and "lockbox") is one
aspect of the phenomenon. This terminology is used to suggest
that Medicare administrators "save" contributions in a "trust
fund," even though CMS either spends the money immediately,
or loans it to the Treasury (which spends the money on other
things) in exchange for a commitment that is binding on future
taxpayers. So much for the purported superior ability of government to balance the interests of future generations against those of
current voters! Politicians display a similarly flexible acquaintance
with the truth when they assert that beneficiaries deserve enhanced
benefits (such as a prescription drug benefit) simply because at
some time in the past they paid some amount into the system.
Such strategies are an invitation to disaster. Indeed, pyramid
schemes such as Medicare self-destruct precisely because everyone
takes out of the pot more than they put in.

One example of the effect of Medicare on political truthfulness
is demonstrated by the whoppers politicians will tell to justify
their attempts to "save" the program from self-destruction or to
extract political advantage from the "reform" proposals of their
opponents. Both Republicans and Democrats know they are
unelectable if they speak candidly about the economic problems
facing Medicare. Accordingly, Republicans package their reform

Medicare's Nonexistent "Trust Fund"

Despite bipartisan references to a Medicare "trust fund," there is, as you know, no such thing. The HI and SMI "trust funds" are actually merely a drawer in CMS headquarters filled with IOUs. In a fit of candor that was quickly corrected, President Clinton's fiscal year 2000 budget analysis accurately described the economic substance of "trust funds":

> These balances are available to finance future benefit payments and other trust fund expenditures—but only in a bookkeeping sense. These funds are not set up to be pension funds, like the funds of private pension plans. They do not consist of real economic assets that can be drawn down in the future to fund benefits. Instead, they are claims on the Treasury that, when redeemed, will have to be financed by raising taxes, borrowing from the public, or reducing benefits or other expenditures. The existence of large trust fund balances, therefore, does not, by itself, have any impact on the Government's ability to pay benefits.[8]

Whether the "trust fund" is empty, or has twice as many IOUs as it does now, has no effect whatsoever on the financial position of the Medicare program.

Simply stated, Medicare's "trust funds" deserve no trust. This simple ruse has allowed us to create public confidence in what is, in reality, a confidence game.

proposals as attempts to "modernize" the Medicare benefit package and offer beneficiaries more options. Democrats focus their efforts on price caps and prayer. Neither approach is likely to produce actuarially balanced and economically sustainable promises to purchasers/investors—the absolute minimum expected of a private insurance plan or investment.

Consider a concrete example. As outlined in chapter 2, Medicare has two parts: Part A, which is paid for with payroll contributions, and Part B, which is paid for with general revenues and beneficiary contributions. Part A has been subject to periodic crises, as the Medicare trustees dutifully announce that the Part A "trust fund" will go bankrupt in a few years. There are only two legitimate strategies to address this problem: increase the flow of revenues into the Part A "trust fund" or decrease the flow of payments out of the Part A "trust fund." Part B provides a seeming "third way"—shifting costs from Part A to Part B. This approach appears to solve the problem but it actually makes it worse by hiding the severity of the problem, and suggesting to people that Medicare's problems can be addressed through sleight of hand.

One recent use of this strategy exemplifies the opportunities for mischief. In 1997, the Clinton administration announced a plan to "save" Medicare. The plan included a broad array of statutory and regulatory changes, the most significant (and least noticed) of which was to transfer home health care from Part A to Part B. For most people, an expenditure is an expenditure, regardless of where the money comes from. Budgeting in the government works differently. Moving home health care out of Part A "saved" Medicare almost $100 billion and extended the life of the "trust fund" even though the same costs were incurred elsewhere in the budget, and they still had to be paid.[9] When asked about this scheme, HHS Secretary Donna Shalala roboti-cally replied that the change was appropriate because it was consistent with the original structural design of Medicare.[10] If Secretary Shalala had actually wanted to revert to the original structure of Medicare, she should have suggested that beneficiaries pay 50 percent of the costs of Part B instead of the current 25 percent—but that suggestion was conspicuously absent from the Clinton administration's budgetary proposal. As you know, the road to hell is paved with such stratagems and rationalizations.

In theory, one could also keep this strategy up indefinitely, and maintain the "trust fund" in surplus simply by transferring out expenses that can no longer be covered by Part A contribu-tions. Of course, this "wishing makes it so" approach to program budgeting only increases the long-term severity of Medicare's fiscal crisis.

To be sure, Medicare affects truthfulness on both sides of the political aisle. The debate over the MMA involved an ever-changing list of numbers calculating the full cost of the benefit, and some evidence that the Bush administration hid from Con-gress what its own actuaries thought the price tag would be. President Bush had promised a bill that would cost no more than $400 billion over the 10-year budget period. A bill that cost much more than that amount would lose too many Republi-can votes to pass (even though it might have picked up votes from Democrats, who wanted a benefit that was more than twice as expensive as the Republicans' ceiling). The administration refused to release its own estimate (by CMS actuaries) of the cost of the MMA, instead relying on a Congressional Budget Office estimate of $395 billion.[11] When the CMS estimate was released two months after the vote on the MMA, it turned out CMS had scored the MMA at $534 billion[12]—a figure almost $140 billion more than Congress had been led to believe.

To be sure, both estimates were plausible, and the differences were the result of differing assumptions—as is often the case with actuarial estimates. However, the dramatically higher price tag precipitated a storm of controversy—compounded when it become known that the head of CMS had warned Medicare's chief actuary that the actuary would face disciplinary action if he responded to congressional inquiries about the estimated cost of the MMA before it was signed into law.

The more general point is that Medicare encourages politicians to ignore or hide the truth, and even gives them the tools to do so. For example, the combination of the 10-year budget horizon and the plasticity of budget estimates created many opportunities for "creative" accounting, and allowed us to push through a budget-busting prescription drug benefit without anyone raising an alarm. Indeed, after its enactment the estimates of the MMA's 10-year cost jumped from $395 billion, to $534 billion, to $690 billion,[13] to $732 billion,[14] to $1.2 trillion.[15] We can be proud that we were able to hide the ball so well for so long—and it will be much harder to repeal the MMA than to enact it, despite its budget-busting consequences. Admittedly, some of the increase in these budgetary estimates is because the early estimates cover a different 10-year window—that is, the early estimates include a phase-in period, while the later estimates assume a fully operational benefit. Whatever the cause, many people feel they were lied to. So, it's all good from our perspective.

Finally, these estimates pertain to the benefit as enacted. There are already numerous proposals to expand the scope of the prescription drug benefit, all tied to its perceived "failings." Thus, what was an unaffordable expansion of an already-unsustainable program has quickly become a "floor" for future negotiations over how quickly our product will grow.

11. The Threat of Exorcism

Of course, we must always be conscious of the threat of exorcism. The seven deadly sins are deeply imbedded within Medicare, but each can be exorcised if there are sufficient political will and popular support to do so. Over the past 40 years, our angelic opponents have repeatedly sought to wrest the Medicare program from our demonic influence—to date without success. Our ability to maintain our winning streak depends on our ability to meet the threat of exorcism head-on, and "demonize" those who advocate responsible reform. The policy proposals that raise the most immediate threat to our plans are as follows.

Demand-Side Conservatism

The principal ideological threat to Medicare is demand-side conservatism, referred to in some circles as the "ownership society."[1] The basic idea driving demand-side conservatism is the hard truth that it is much more difficult to reduce the supply of government than it is to reduce the demand for government. Reducing the supply of government requires visible cutting of programs and personnel—and each program typically has a constituency that will fight viciously for its continuation.

Conversely, demand-side conservatism shrinks the demand for government by empowering individual citizens to make their own decisions, and making them more self-reliant and responsible, and less dependent on government. As one commentator put it, "With individuals allowed to decide how to save, invest and handle their

---

**Government Programs Don't Die—
or Even Fade Away**

Pick a program, any program. How about the strategic helium reserve? In 1925, a federal law put the government in the business of ensuring that an adequate supply of helium was available to fill the blimps that were viewed as a vital part of American military power. More than 80 years later, and after the invention of the jet engine, guess who is still operating a strategic helium reserve? The sad saga of mohair subsidies is another illustration of this phenomenon. Those payouts were created in 1954 to ensure that enough wool was available to make military uniforms. The program was finally eliminated in 1994, only to be resurrected in 1999. (Let's not even mention the excise tax on long-distance phone calls, enacted in 1898 to fund the Spanish-American War and finally terminated in 2006 after the IRS kept losing cases in court.)

---

health-care expenses, they'd demand less from government."[2] If citizens demand less from government, it will erode support for the Medicare program, and the ideological foundation on which the program is built. We anticipate our foes will employ four distinct strategies to push demand-side conservatism.

Means Testing

As noted earlier, the MMA allowed means testing in Medicare for the first time. Some very wealthy seniors will be required to pay a larger share of the cost of their Part B coverage, whereas most seniors will pay more for their Part D coverage than low-income seniors. If Medicare were wholly means-tested, it would be instantly transformed into a program for poor seniors, instead of one for the poor, the wealthy, and everyone in between. Once the Medicare program does not include all the elderly, it becomes much easier for legislators to impose significant funding and benefit cuts, and the political punch of pro-Medicare demagoguery becomes much less powerful when all that is at stake is the health and welfare of poor people. If that happens, it will be much harder for us to meet the financial projections outlined in your original plan—and that would dramatically slow our timetable for destroying the American Republic. To date, we have been successful at resisting any broad-based attempt to means-test the Medicare program, although we should remain on our demonic guard against further efforts by the enemy.

Defined Contributions

The biggest change in private pensions over the past 40 years has been the move from defined benefit to defined contribution plans. Defined benefit plans represent a promise by the employer to provide a certain level of benefits over the course of retirement. Conversely, defined contribution plans represent a promise by the employer to contribute a certain amount of money toward financing retirement benefits for the employee.

In most important respects, Medicare is a defined benefit plan, since it has agreed to provide all necessary medical care to its beneficiaries—regardless of cost or cost-effectiveness. Switching Medicare to a defined contribution approach, where each beneficiary would receive a set amount of funds (or a set percentage of the average premium) with which to purchase health care coverage (or whatever else they wanted, if it was structured as a cash-based voucher program), would instantly change the dynamics of the federal budgeting process. Beneficiaries would suddenly be spending their own money on health care services, instead of everyone else's. Congress would get out of the business of micromanaging payment formulas and benefits. The combination of responsible medical consumption by beneficiaries plus intense competition between providers to deliver high-quality, cost-effective care would be disastrous for our plans.

Of course, the Medicare program would still face various financing risks associated with demographic changes, and there would be political debates over the amount of the voucher, but the annual cost of the program would be under direct congressional control. Congress would be forced to decide each year how much they were willing to spend on the Medicare program. Instead of an open-ended pyramid scheme, Medicare would be in the business of offering vouchers so that beneficiaries could purchase their own coverage. We succeeded in killing this dangerous proposal when it was recommended in 1999 by a bipartisan Medicare Commission, and we intend to use the same tactics for all such future initiatives.

Private Contracting

In the mid-1990s, we grew concerned about the risk that Medicare beneficiaries would privately contract with providers for Medicare-covered services, either to protect their privacy or because they wanted to pay more to obtain certain treatments not otherwise available to Medicare beneficiaries. Such contracts could easily undermine Medicare's monopoly power and help create true market competition—which would devastate our plans. We pushed for a law that would kill such contracts without quite saying so, and we were successful in getting a provision that allowed such contracts only if the provider agreed not to treat any Medicare patients for two years.[3] Since most providers can't afford to do without Medicare payments for two years, this provision effectively killed the private contracting market. We anticipate that our enemies will attempt to revisit this issue in the coming years, and we will continue to make every effort to hold them off.

Health Savings Accounts

Health savings accounts (HSAs) represent the most direct application of demand-side conservatism to health care. HSAs allow people to pay for current health care expenditures and save for future health care expenditures using a tax-advantaged savings account and a high-deductible health plan. Like a defined contribution plan, HSAs create a direct economic incentive for consumers to make cost-benefit tradeoffs in their health care consumption decisions. Of course, once the deductible is exceeded, the incentives change, unless there is significant cost sharing in the high-deductible health plan.

Although Medicare beneficiaries do not qualify for HSAs, there have been repeated attempts to enroll Medicare beneficiaries in similar plans, called medical savings accounts. We have thus far held these efforts at bay.[4] The long-term effect of HSAs, however, will be to reduce the demand for Medicare, since beneficiaries will not need government coverage if they have sufficient tax-advantaged savings and can tap into a robust coverage market for a high-deductible health plan. We saw this problem coming, and were successful in restricting HSAs in the Health Insurance Portability and Accountability Act of 1996. Unfortunately, those restrictions were eliminated by the MMA, and now there are more than three million Americans with such coverage, and proposals to expand HSAs further. We expect that HSAs will pose a continuing problem for us.

Repeal of the Medicare Drug Program

Although the MMA included HSAs, we ultimately decided to back it because, as described previously, the prescription drug benefit simultaneously allowed us to worsen the financial outlook for the Medicare program dramatically and raise the partisan stakes for future reforms. Yet, there is always the risk that the ballooning cost of Part D may encourage Congress to repeal the prescription drug benefits, while leaving in place the HSAs. It is unclear whether the rollout of the program has caused sufficient discontent among senior citizens to drive a mass movement in favor of repeal, although there are some early indications of dissatisfaction. We should be vigilant in our efforts to ensure that Part D stays in its current form.

Greater Competition

Medicare embodies a big-government command-and-control approach to paying for health care services, and the U.S. health care system looks the way that it does because it was built around incentives created by Medicare. On the other hand, the broader market for health care services is much more dynamic, with constant innovation in service delivery forms.[5] Competition from new entrants can disrupt the cozy cartel we have created by buying off incumbent providers. Market entry also disrupts the cross-subsidies we have built into the system. These cross-subsidies help make insurance unaffordable to many working Americans. The creative destruction that results from competition and market entry obviously threatens the way in which we have always done business.

For example, physician-owned single-specialty hospitals have emerged in recent years. Most of these single-specialty hospitals focus on providing care to patients with cardiac and orthopedic conditions. Obviously, these new entrants pose a risk to our long-standing partners in the community hospital sector (while also exploiting the gluttony of physician-investors). Although the incentive to open a specialty hospital is driven, in part, by Medicare "overpayment" for cardiac and orthopedic services, we opted not to fix that problem, but instead secured a moratorium on Medicare reimbursement of specialty hospitals. Specialty hospitals are merely the latest manifestation of the threat posed to our plans by market forces.

We also rely on our lobbyists on K Street and in major universities to bleat endlessly about market failures in health care, and claim that these market failures justify government taking steps that eliminate competition. As you well know, and as Judge Frank Easterbrook observed with alarming prescience, we "are concerned not about market failures but about market successes— about the prospect that the sort of world people prefer when they vote with their own pocketbooks will depart from the proposers' ideas of what people *ought* to prefer. Next thing you know, why, economic transactions between consenting adults will break out *right in public view!*"[6] Since we can't have that, we will continue to use Medicare aggressively to frustrate consumer preferences.

Prudent Purchasing

Provider participation in Medicare (and provider support for the program) is dependent on it interfering as little as possible with the autonomy of individual providers. As such, if Medicare ever stops being a passive payer of bills, and starts acting like a prudent purchaser, it will destroy the coalition of provider-supporters we have painstakingly built for the program. As a prophylactic measure to address this risk, we hard-wired a considerable degree of passivity into the Medicare program (making it "a feature, not a bug," as they say in computer circles). As noted previously, the enabling legislation placed major limitations on the ability of program administrators to exercise any real oversight over quality or volume, and delegated responsibility for claims processing to program vendors. As also noted previously, we compounded this passivity by using administrators from the SSA to run the program for the first 12 years.

Tom Scully, the former head of CMS, nicely summarized the consequences of this purchasing structure on Medicare's operations:

> [Medicare should be able to] say to a caregiver, "Look, you are a rotten provider. You are not a good provider. You are a low-quality provider. We are going to pay you differentially." The flaw of the fee-for-service system is that it has to pay every provider the same amount in every community. As soon as that common payment is the law, the program inevitably will be a disaster.[7]

Even Medicare's enthusiasts acknowledge that because it is an open-ended defined-benefit program, "there is no practical means of controlling the volume of services billed to the program, let alone to assess the medical and economic merits of these services."[8]

The degree to which Medicare does not employ prudent purchasing techniques is best demonstrated by juxtaposing Medicare with purchasing everywhere else in the economy—including other government purchasing. Al Dunlap, former president of Scott Paper and Sunbeam, provides a useful list of purchasing techniques that he believes any company should use in buying anything.[9]

1. Leverage volume as much as possible.
2. Narrow suppliers to a handful.
3. Encourage multiple vendors to bid on requirements.
4. Negotiate hard contracts.
5. Practice brinkmanship. Let vendors know that they don't have an eternal lock on your business.
6. Significantly challenge the procurement organization to take cost out and support them in doing so.
7. Ask vendors to help reduce costs by utilizing their own expertise and resources.

The striking thing is that Medicare has historically done none of these things! Although Medicare is currently attempting to implement pay-for-performance, it has thankfully, taken only baby steps in that direction. We will continue to resist pay-for-performance and seek to minimize the amount of money that is tied to the attainment of objective benchmarks of quality.

To be sure, these risks are not new. We faced them at the outset of the Medicare program, and we must be vigilant to ensure that Medicare's purchasing power does not become a force for good in the health care marketplace.

The "45-Percent Trigger"

The final threat to our plans is not really a threat in itself, but could prove nettlesome by giving our opponents an opportunity to educate the American public about Medicare. As you know, illumination can only add to public support for exorcism.

The MMA requires Medicare's trustees to report each year whether, at any time over the subsequent seven years, 45 percent

When Medicare's Purchasing Power
Is Used as a Force for Good

We have largely succeeded in killing the efforts of our angelic opponents to hijack the Medicare program's purchasing power to improve the health care marketplace, with one important exception. When Medicare was started, the Civil Rights Act of 1964 (another of our failings) flatly prohibited segregated hospitals from being included in the Medicare program.

We were faced with two unappetizing options. If we pushed ahead with Medicare, the countless demon-hours we had spent creating and maintaining racial segregation would be swept away in the health care sector almost overnight—and the desegregation of hospitals would make it easier for our angelic opponents to move against other forms of racial segregation. On the other hand, if we held the line on segregation, the Medicare program would almost certainly fail at the outset, at least in the poorest Southern states in the heart of the Confederacy.

You ultimately decided that we would put our bets on Medicare instead of segregation, but ever since, we have been extremely careful to ensure that Medicare just processes the paperwork and shovels money out the door to providers, irrespective of the quality of the services they provide, or the medical necessity for those services. We do not believe the recent efforts to create pay-for-performance in Medicare will impede our efforts, since the financial stakes are far too small to affect even the worst-quality provider.

or more of Medicare spending will come from general tax revenues (as opposed to dedicated revenue sources such as the Medicare payroll tax or beneficiary premiums). If the trustees make such a determination two years in a row, that triggers a "Medicare funding warning" that the trustees must send to the president. The MMA states that when the trustees pull that trigger, the president must propose legislation to keep the share of Medicare spending that comes from general revenues below 45 percent of overall Medicare spending. The MMA further states that Congress must consider the proposed legislation on an expedited basis.

By itself, that "Medicare funding warning" is a pathetic response to the ever-worsening financial picture of Medicare. To comply, the president could propose to increase Medicare taxes, increase beneficiary premiums, cut benefits, or reform the program. All well and good. However, Congress is under no obligation to do anything at all. If it wished, Congress could respond to the president's proposal by *increasing* Medicare spending! This "45-percent trigger" is the equivalent of having the fire department periodically update you on how much of your house has been consumed by flames—and propose ways to slow (or even to hasten) the burn—rather than just put the fire out.

Yet the "45-percent trigger" does pose a potential threat. In their 2006 report, Medicare's trustees made the first of the required two determinations. Many observers believe they will make the second such determination in 2007. If so, the resulting "Medicare funding warning" may create a teachable moment where our enemies could educate the public about just how much of their fiscal house we have already consumed in flames. If they are successful in doing that, our enemies may even be able to enact one or more of the reforms mentioned in this chapter as early as 2007. To prevent that calamity, we will encourage our allies to assert that the 45-percent threshold is an artificial and arbitrary limit to impose on general revenue financing. That riposte has the benefit of being true, even while it hides our true purpose.

Summary

Although we face a number of threats, our plans for Medicare are going well. Legislative inertia helps ensure that things will remain as they are—steadily worsening for the American Republic, and getting better every day for us. We believe the most likely threat to materialize is a renewed effort to move to a defined contribution (premium support) model, similar to that proposed by the 1999 Medicare Commission. We believe the new Medicare Commission proposed by President George W. Bush is likely to end up proposing something similar. However, unless our enemies in the celestial regions get their act together, we believe we will be able to prevent this initiative from getting very far. As we both know, our nemesis only helps those who help themselves—and we are well positioned to discourage any of that.

The other threats to our plans are real, but with one exception they nibble at the margins of our plans, or have a time frame that will not interfere with our schedule. The exception is the threat to repeal Part D—which we should take very seriously.

12. Conclusion

It has been said that your greatest achievement was to convince the world that Your Eminence does not exist.[1] You have built on that feat by creating a government program that serves all of our ends, but whose defenders believe serves those of our enemies. Medicare pits the young against the old; pits providers against lawyers against politicians against bureaucrats; and sets providers against one another. Your design of this program guarantees that politicians will make promises they cannot keep and delays the day of reckoning so that the citizenry will order their entire lives around the unreasonable expectations the politicians create. You have guaranteed that when the day of reckoning finally arrives, all you-know-what will break loose. You have freed the self-interest of these mortals from its natural restraints. As a result, the seven deadly sins have blossomed, as have our accounts.

The achievements outlined in this report are even more noteworthy given the considerable skepticism with which Americans have historically regarded government-run anything—and their repeated rejection of government-run health care proposals throughout the 20th century. Consider the fate of the Clinton administration's proposal for universal health care. Notwithstanding initial favorable press coverage, the Clinton plan suffered substantial decreases in public support as its details became clear. It was obvious that it had passed the tipping point when bumper stickers appeared announcing "National Health Care?—The compassion of the IRS!—The efficiency of the post office!—All at Pentagon prices!"[2] Of course, once we completely take over the American Republic, we will be able to address such impertinence directly and decisively, instead of relying on our contacts in the media to spread our message.

All of the building blocks are in place for our plans to destabilize the American Republic. Although actuarial estimates vary somewhat (regrettably, we have not succeeded in suborning all the actuaries), the Medicare budget is heading for a demographic brick wall at an accelerating rate. Every attempt to impose fiscal discipline triggers squeals of outrage from affected providers, beneficiary groups, and true believers in this "sacred" intergenerational pyramid scheme. To date, we have forestalled every attempt to reform Medicare in any meaningful way, and we are reasonably confident that we will be able to do so in the future—unless of course the threats outlined in chapter 11 come to fruition. We should devote our best efforts to ensure that they do not.

Absent true reform, our best calculation is that the Medicare program will completely implode within two generations. Incremental efforts to "fix" Medicare will extend the process only slightly, while simultaneously breeding dissension and class warfare—confirming the predictions outlined in your original memo. As long as no one learns of our plans, we look forward to an ever-increasing U.S. market share. Best of all, we obtain this increase in market share without any further promotional or recruiting expenditures. You have replaced the virtuous circle at the heart of the American Republic with a vicious circle.[3] All of us in the North American Division of DISS bow our horns in awe of your subtle genius.

> Have a hellish day,
> Underling Demon 666
> DASCAR
> DISS

PART II

EPILOGUE

13. A Sacred Bond between the Generations?

Of course, it is libelous to suggest that the most successful program of Johnson's Great Society is a demonic plot. However, satire provides a tool for exploring some of Medicare's problems in a less confrontational manner than would otherwise be the case. At least that's my story and I'm sticking to it.

To be sure, many of Medicare's defenders react to even the slightest criticism of their favorite program with a ferocity that demonstrates that their enthusiasm has more to do with ideology than the actuarially sound/goo-goo approach they would insist on if we were talking about anything other than Medicare. Imagine the cries of righteous indignation that we would hear from Medicare's defenders if Congress established a program with similar spending projections and unimpressive quality to secure weapons for the military.

Satire thus has the potential to provoke the program's defenders to at least acknowledge some of Medicare's problems. Of course, it would be foolish to be overly optimistic about how much of Medicare's reality its defenders are likely to acknowledge. Indeed, it is likely they will get stuck at either denial (stage one) or anger (stage two), instead of progressing to bargaining (stage three) or depression (stage four)—let alone acceptance (stage five).[1]

Consider what happened when I presented some considerably less pointed remarks at the conference at Washington and Lee University School of Law. One of Medicare's most enthusiastic supporters responded by making an impassioned speech that it was improper to describe Medicare as a "Ponzi scheme," and the program should not be judged by the standards that would apply to a private pension because it was actually a "sacred bond" between the generations. (Leave aside the fact that I never used the word "Ponzi" in my remarks. I did note that the Medicare program bore certain similarities to an intergenerational pyramid scheme, which is something quite different. Of course, it is possible that the use of this term by the commentator was a Freudian slip.) His words brought enthusiastic applause from those members of the audience who had heard enough bad news of the sort found in this book and were more than ready to ignore Medicare's problems on the basis of empty political sloganeering.

Yet, this "explanation" provides no basis for believing that Medicare should not be judged by the standards of any other government expenditure or private investment—let alone a defensible theory for understanding how any given act of one Congress magically becomes a "sacred bond between the generations." Instead, this "explanation" is, at best, nothing more than an exercise in sophistry and, at worst, simply another example of the "wishing makes it so" approach to Medicare that is characteristic of the program's more vehement defenders.

If Medicare really were a sacred bond between the generations, Medicare reform would not be a live issue on the political agenda—which it has been for the past decade. There would not have been a bipartisan commission on Medicare reform issuing a report in 1999—which there was—let alone another bipartisan commission on Medicare reform gearing up as this book goes to press—which there is. The 1999 bipartisan commission would not have considered moving the program from a defined benefit to a defined contribution approach—which it did. A clear majority of the commission would not have voted for this approach—

which they did. There would not have been proposals to means-test Part B premiums in 1993, 1995, and 1997—which there were. Nor would the MMA have imposed means testing of Part B premiums—which it did. There wouldn't be a host of bipartisan initiatives to make Medicare a more prudent purchaser of health care services—which there are. Stated bluntly, Medicare reform is a live issue because Medicare is *not* a sacred bond between the generations. It's just a program and a pretty mediocre one at that.

The depth and sincerity of Medicare defenders' faith in the program (and in centralized command-and-control administered pricing systems more generally) should not obscure the reality that Medicare's philosophical foundations are contested and up for reconsideration to a degree not seen since its enactment. Given this scrutiny, it is worth considering how Medicare fares in light of the parable that Milton Friedman told when he was honored for lifetime achievement at the White House on May 9, 2002:

> My views on government spending can be summarized by the following parable. If you spend your own money on yourself, you are very concerned about how much is spent and how it is spent. If you spend your own money on someone else, you are still very much concerned about how much is spent, but somewhat less concerned about how it is spent. If you spend someone else's money on yourself, you are not too concerned about how much is spent, but you are very concerned about how it is spent. However, if you spend someone else's money on someone else, you are not very concerned about how much is spent or how it is spent.[2]

Three guesses as to which of the four formulations best describes Medicare—although one's answer does depend on one's position on the political spectrum and on whether one is currently a Medicare beneficiary or provider of services to the same. Of course, it is possible that Friedman's insight has nothing to do with the debate over Medicare and the preferences of Medicare's supporters. It is also possible that the moon is made of green cheese.

Despite this reality, there is still considerable reluctance in Washington to face the dire facts about Medicare's actual performance. Consider what happened when a draft copy of this book was sent to the office of a prominent senator by my editor, with a request for a "blurb." My editor was told that even though the book was "useful . . . our health policy director won't let us blurb it and . . . won't read it either for that matter," because the book is critical of the new Medicare prescription drug benefit. Evidently, it may take more than satire to get reformers to acknowledge Medicare's problems.

Finally, during the symposium at which this work was first presented, one of the commentators described Medicare as a flower-child remnant of the 1960s. I responded that it was the only flower child I was aware of with more than $340 billion per year with which to fix prices and screw up the market for health care services. A more devastating comeback escaped me at the time, but occurred to me later. In the first *Austin Powers* film, the movie ends with a confrontation between the film's hero (Powers) and its villain (Dr. Evil). Powers tries to rationalize away the excesses and self-indulgence of the 1960s. Dr. Evil listens to Powers for as long as he can stand it, and finally retorts, "There's nothing more pathetic than an aging hipster."[3]

Herbert Stein, the chairman of President Nixon's Council of Economic Advisers, coined Stein's law: "If something cannot go on forever, it will stop."[4] Medicare's trajectory can't go on forever, and it will have to stop. The only question is when and how. There are better and worse ways to handle the transition to a program that we can actually afford. It is my modest hope that this book will help lead us toward the former, while offering a new villain that can be conveniently blamed for the mess in which we find ourselves.

Time is short, and the longer we delay, the worse our predicament. The basic problem with Medicare is that we find ourselves in a hole, but our collective response seems to be to keep digging. Switching the focus from demons to saints, when it comes to fixing Medicare, we can no longer afford the approach of Saint Augustine, who prayed for chastity and continence, "but not yet."

Appendix A: Glossary

administrative cost: The cost of managing the financing and delivery of health care, including but not limited to billing, claims processing, marketing, profit, and overhead.

catastrophic coverage: Insurance that pays for very large health care expenses.

Centers for Medicare & Medicaid Services (CMS): Part of the U.S. Department of Health and Human Services, CMS is the federal government agency that administers Medicare and Medicaid. It was created in 1977 as the Health Care Financing Administration, and renamed CMS in 2001.

charity care: Free health care given by doctors, nurses, and hospitals.

copayment: A fee that must be paid by patients when they receive health care services.

cost sharing: Requiring the patient to bear some of the cost of treatment. The theory of cost sharing is that it discourages the patient from receiving treatment that is unnecessary or noncostworthy. However, it can also discourage the patient from receiving medically necessary treatment. Cost sharing comes in numerous varieties, including deductibles and copayments.

deductible: The amount a patient must pay out-of-pocket before health insurance will provide coverage.

diagnosis-related groups (DRGs): A payment system adopted by Medicare in 1982. Payments for inpatient hospitalizations are prospectively determined, based on the discharge diagnosis, independent of the actual cost of treatment.

entitlements: A government benefit that is automatically conferred on beneficiaries as a matter of right. The government is required to cover the cost of such benefits, irrespective of their cost. Examples include Social Security and Medicare.

fee for service: A system of paying for professional services on a piecework basis.

formula fight: A dispute as to how the benefits of a particular program should be distributed. At the federal level, a program can distribute radically different amounts to each state, depending on the parameters used to determine the amount distributed. For example, a program that distributes funds based on population will result in different payments than one that gives equal shares to each state, or one that gives equal amounts per hospital, or one that gives equal amounts per square mile within the state boundaries, or . . .

Health Care Financing Administration (HCFA): see **Centers for Medicare & Medicaid Services**.

Health Maintenance Organization (HMO): A prepaid medical care plan. The HMO is paid a fixed amount per patient per month to provide all necessary care.

health savings accounts: Analogous to individual retirement accounts, but employers and employees can make tax-deferred contributions and employees can withdraw funds tax-free to pay covered medical expenses.

long-term care: Generally, care provided by a nursing home.

malpractice: Treatment that fails to meet professional standards of care and results in harm to the patient.

managed care: Refers to a diverse array of arrangements designed to lower the cost and improve the quality of health care services, by restricting the choices of both patient and provider.

means testing: Allowing an individual to be the beneficiary of a government program only if they "need" the benefit—that is, if they don't have the means to provide for themselves. Means testing generally excludes potential beneficiaries that exceed a specified level of income or assets. Medicare is generally not means tested.

Medicaid: The federal social insurance entitlement program created in 1965 to provide medical care to the poor. Medicaid is means tested.

medical savings accounts: see **health savings accounts**.

Medicare: The federal social insurance entitlement program enacted in 1965 to provide medical care to the elderly and disabled.

Medicare Catastrophic Coverage Act: This law was passed by Congress in 1988. It covered Medicare beneficiaries with catastrophic medical expenses, capped out-of-pocket expenses, and covered prescription drugs. It did not cover long-term care, and the costs of the benefits were imposed on senior citizens, with higher premiums paid by those with larger incomes. After many senior citizens objected, Congress repealed the law in 1989.

Part A: The portion of the Medicare program that pays for inpatient hospitalization. Also known as hospital insurance.

Part B: The portion of the Medicare program that pays for outpatient treatment and treatment by physicians. Also known as supplementary medical insurance.

Part C: The managed care option in Medicare. Previously referred to as Medicare + Choice; now called Medicare Advantage.

Part D: The newest portion of the Medicare program that pays for prescription drugs for those who enroll.

premium support: A proposal to reform Medicare that would provide Medicare beneficiaries with vouchers that they would use to purchase medical insurance. The amount of the voucher would vary, depending on the cost of providing coverage for the particular beneficiary. The proposal was endorsed by a majority of the 1999 Medicare Reform Commission, chaired by then-Senator John Breaux (D-LA) and Representative Bill Thomas (R-CA).

prospective payment system (PPS): The system used by Medicare to pay for inpatient hospitalizations. See **diagnosis-related groups**.

rent seeking: The process of profiting through manipulation of government regulations, generally at the expense of consumers and competitors.

Resource-Based Relative Value Scale (RBRVS): The RBRVS was enacted in 1992 as a way of systematizing Medicare payments for physician services. Several criteria are used to rank the complexity and difficulty of performing each specified service. A conversion factor translates that figure into a specific dollar amount that is paid for each service.

seven deadly sins: Avarice, gluttony, envy, sloth, lust, anger, and vanity.

social insurance: A government program where everyone is taxed to provide benefits to those who qualify as beneficiaries.

Appendix B: Abbreviations and Acronyms

AMA	American Medical Association
CMS	Centers for Medicare and Medicaid Services
DASCAR	Deputy Assistant Special Coordinator for Accelerating Recruitment
DISS	Department of Illness and Satanic Services
DRG	diagnosis related group
FCA	False Claims Act
HCFA	Health Care Financing Administration
HHS	Health and Human Services, Department of
HI	hospital insurance (Part A of Medicare)
HSA	health savings account
MMA	Medicare Prescription Drug Improvement and Modernization Act of 2003 (also known as the Medicare Modernization Act)
PPS	prospective payment system
RBRVS	Resource-Based Relative Value Scale
SMI	supplementary medical insurance (Part B of Medicare)
SSA	Social Security Administration

Appendix C: Background Information on Medicare Parts A–D

Part A covers hospital stays, including the cost of a semiprivate room, meals, regular nursing services, operating and recovery rooms, intensive care, inpatient prescription drugs, laboratory tests, x-rays, and other medically necessary services and supplies provided in the hospital. Part A covers stays in general hospitals, psychiatric hospitals, inpatient rehabilitation, and long-term care hospitalization when medically necessary. Part A will also pay for some nursing home stays if they occur within a certain amount of time after a hospital stay. Part A also covers some limited home health care costs if they follow a hospital or nursing home stay. Finally, hospice care is available for beneficiaries with life expectancies of six months or less who elect to forgo the standard Medicare benefits for treatment of their illness and to receive only hospice care for it.

Part B covers outpatient medical services, including services provided by physicians, chiropractors, podiatrists, dentists, optometrists, clinical psychologists, physician assistants, and nurse practitioners. Part B also covers visits to an emergency room, outpatient clinic, and ambulatory surgery center; ambulance services; most physical and occupational therapy and speech pathology services; most home health care not covered under Part A; laboratory tests, x-rays and other diagnostic radiology services; some preventive care screening tests; approved durable medical equipment (oxygen tanks, wheelchairs, and prosthetic devices); radiation therapy; renal (kidney) dialysis and transplants; heart, lung, heart-lung, liver, pancreas, and bone marrow transplants; intestinal transplants; and drugs that cannot be self-administered.

Beneficiaries enrolled in both Part A and Part B can instead choose to participate in a Medicare Advantage plan through Part C. Parts A and B are the province of fee-for-service health care, while Part C is the managed care option. Medicare Advantage plans include HMOs, provider-sponsored organizations, and preferred provider organizations. Medicare Advantage plans are required to provide at least the current Medicare benefit package, excluding hospice services. Plans may offer additional covered services. There has been considerable turbulence in Medicare Part C, as managed care organizations have elected not to continue in the program. Currently, approximately 15 percent of Medicare beneficiaries are in a Medicare Advantage plan.

Part D currently provides subsidized access to prescription drug coverage for those who elect to participate. Beneficiaries may enroll in either a stand-alone prescription drug plan or an integrated Medicare Advantage plan that offers Part D coverage. Part D includes most Food and Drug Administration–approved prescription drugs and biologicals. Plans may set up formularies for their prescription drug coverage, subject to certain statutory standards. Part D also provides heavy subsidies to employers who offer similar prescription drug coverage to their retirees.

Recommended Reading

The following books offer a diverse array of perspectives on Medicare. In different ways, they each complement the analysis contained in this book. Those who are interested in reading further are directed to any of the books below.

Blevins, Sue A. *Medicare's Midlife Crisis.* Washington: Cato Institute, 2001.

Jost, Timothy S. *Disentitlement? The Threats Facing Our Public Health-Care Programs and a Rights-Based Response.* New York: Oxford University Press, 2003.

Marmor, Theodore. *The Politics of Medicare.* 2nd ed. New York: Aldine De Gruyter, 2000.

Moon, Marilyn. *Medicare Now and in the Future.* 2nd ed. Washington: Urban Institute Press.

Oberlander, Jon A. *The Political Life of Medicare.* Chicago: University of Chicago Press, 2003.

Rettenmaier, Andrew J., and Thomas R. Saving. *The Economics of Medicare Reform.* Kalamazoo, MI: W. E. Upjohn Institute for Employment Research, 2000.

Notes

Front Matter

1. See Stephen Vincent Benet, *The Devil and Daniel Webster* (New York: Rinehart and Company, Inc., 1937); C. S. Lewis, *The Screwtape Letters* (San Francisco: Harpers, 2001); Uwe Reinhardt, "The Predictable Managed Care Kvetch on the Rocky Road from Adolescence to Adulthood," *Journal of Health Policy Politics and Law* 24 (1999): 897; Mark Twain, *A Connecticut Yankee in King Arthur's Court* (Oxford: Oxford University Press, 1996).

2. Uwe E. Reinhardt, "Healthcare Crisis: Who's at Risk?" *PBS.org.*, November 3, 2000, http://www.pbs.org/healthcarecrisis/Exprts_intrvw/u_reinhardt.htm. See also Uwe E. Reinhardt, "How the Devil Subverted the Nation's Soul: An Allegory about American Health Policy," in *Social Insurance Issues for the Nineties: Proceedings of the Third Conference of the National Academy of Social Insurance* (Debuque, IA: Kandell Hunt, 1992), pp. 79–93.

Introduction

1. Mark Twain, introduction to *The Adventures of Huckleberry Finn* (New York: Harper and Brothers, 1901).

Chapter 1

1. Pope St. Gregory the Great, *Moralia in Job (595)*, XXXI, cap. xlv.

2. Benet, *Devil and Daniel Webster*.

3. Satan, *Destabilizing the American Republic with a Government-Mandated Intergenerational Pyramid Scheme* (Brimstoneware Press, 1964) (generally unavailable, at least in this life).

4. Benet, *Devil and Daniel Webster*.

5. *United States ex rel. Gerald Mayo v. Satan and His Staff*, 54 F.R.D. 282 (W.D. Pa. 1971).

Chapter 2

1. Eric Patachnik and Julian Zelizer, "Paying for Medicare: Benefits, Budgets, and Wilbur Mill's Policy Legacy," *Journal of Health Politics, Policy and Law* 26 (1987): 7–36.

2. "President Lyndon B. Johnson's Remarks with President Truman at the Signing in Independence of the Medicare Bill, July 30, 1965," http://www.lbjlib.utexas.edu/johnson/archives.hom/speeches.hom/650730.asp.

3. Robert M. Ball, "What Medicare Architects Had in Mind," *Health Affairs* 14 (Winter 1995): 62–73.

4. "Medicare Fact Sheet: Medicare Spending and Financing," Kaiser Family Foundation, April 2005, p. 2, http://www.kff.org/medicare/upload/7305.pdf.

5. Mark Pauly, "Means Testing in Medicare," *Health Affairs Web Exclusive*, December 8, 2004, pp. W4-546–W4-557, http://content.healthaffairs.org/cgi/reprint/hlthaff.w4.546v1.pdf.

6. Michael Cannon and Michael Tanner, *Healthy Competition: What's Holding Back Health Care and How to Free It* (Washington: Cato Institute, 2005), pp. 91–103. See also Stephen A. Moses, "Aging America's Achilles' Heel: Medicaid Long-Term Care," Cato Institute Policy Analysis no. 549, September 1, 2005.

7. Sue A. Blevins, *Medicare's Midlife Crisis* (Washington: Cato Institute, 2001), pp. 45–46.

8. Stephen Heffler et al., "U.S. Health Spending Projections for 2004–2014," *Health Affairs Web Exclusive*, February 23, 2005, p. w5-78, http://content.healthaffairs.org/cgi/reprint/hlthaff.w5.74v1.pdf.

9. U.S. Bureau of the Census, *The 2006 Statistical Abstract: The National Data Book* (Washington: Government Printing Office, 2006), Table 149.

10. "Remarks by HHS Secretary Tommy G. Thompson at Press Conference Announcing Reforming Medicare and Medicaid Agency," U.S. Department of Health and Human Services, June 14, 2001, http://www.hhs.gov/news/press/2001pres/20010614b.html.

11. See Statement of CMS Administrator Thomas Scully, *Health Care and Competition Law and Policy: Hearings before the FTC and DOJ*, Feb. 26, 2003, http://www.ftc.gov/ogc/healthcarehearings/030226trans.pdf.

12. Robert Pear, "Medicare Agency Changes Name in an Effort to Emphasize Services," *New York Times,* June 15, 2001, p. A26.

13. Amy Goldstein, "Health Insurance Agency Gets New Name, Structure," *Washington Post,* June 15, 2001, p. A31.

14. Ellen Nakashima and Ceci Connolly, "Wanted: A HCFA by Any Other Name," *Washington Post,* June 12, 2001, p. A23.

15. Cannon and Tanner, *Healthy Competition,* pp. 72–75; Uwe Reinhardt, "The Medicare World from Both Sides: A Conversation with Tom Scully," *Health Affairs* 22 (Nov.–Dec. 2003): 168.

16. Cannon and Tanner, *Healthy Competition,* p. 51 (see note 6).

17. Clair Snyder and Gerard Anderson, "Do Quality Improvement Organizations Improve the Quality of Hospital Care for Medicare Beneficiaries?" *Journal of the American Medical Association* 293 (2005): 2900.

18. Stephen F. Jencks et al., "Change in the Quality of Care Delivered to Medicare Beneficiaries, 1998–1999 to 2000–2001," *Journal of the American Medical Association* 289 (2003): 305–7.

19. John E. Wennberg et al., "Use of Hospitals, Physician Visits, and Hospice Care during Last Six Months of Life among Cohorts Loyal to Highly Respected Hospitals in the United States," *BMJ* 328 (2004): 607–10.

20. Dartmouth Atlas of Health Care, http://www.dartmouthatlas.org/.

21. James N. Weinstein et al., "Trends and Geographic Variations in Major Surgery for Degenerative Diseases of the Hip, Knee, and Spine" *Health Affairs Web Exclusive* (2004).

22. Elliot S. Fisher et al., "The Implication of Regional Variations in Medicare Spending Part 2: Health Outcomes and Satisfaction with Care," *Annals of Internal Medicine* 138 (2003): 288.

23. Ibid.

24. Katherine Baicker and Amitabh Chandra, "Medicare Spending, the Physician Workforce, and Beneficiaries' Quality of Care," *Health Affairs Web Exclusive,* April 7, 2004, p. W4–187, http://content.healthaffairs.org/cgi/reprint/hlthaff.w4.184v1.pdf.

25. Merrill Matthews, "Medicare's Hidden Administrative Costs: A Comparison of Medicare and the Private Sector," January 10, 2006, http://www.cahi.org/cahi_contents/resources/pdf/CAHI_Medicare_Admin_ Final_ Publication.pdf.

26. David A. Hyman, "Health Care Fraud and Abuse: Market Change Social Norms and 'the Trust Reposed in the Workmen,'" *Journal of Legal Studies* 30 (2001): 531–69.

27. U.S. General Accounting Office, "High Risk Series: An Update (Repeat No. 03-119)," 2003, http://www.gao.gov/pas/2003/d03119.pdf.

28. David A. Hyman, "Does Quality of Care Matter to Medicare?" *Perspectives in Biology and Medicine*, Winter 2003, pp. 55–68.

Chapter 3

1. Theodore Marmor, *The Politics of Medicare*, 2nd ed. (New York: Aldine De Gruyter, 2000), pp. 17–21, 38–41; Paul Starr, *The Social Transformation of American Medicine*, (New York: Basic Books, 1982).

2. Max J. Skidmore, *Medicare and the American Rhetoric of Reconciliation* (Tuscaloosa: University of Alabama Press, 1970), pp. 123–8.

3. James Boswell, *Life of Samuel Johnson*, vol. 8, chap. 2 (London, 1835).

4. Bruce Vladeck, "'The Political Economy of Medicare," *Health Affairs* 18 (1999): 22.

5. Ibid.

6. David A. Hyman and Charles Silver, "You Get What You Pay For: Result-Based Compensation for Health Care," *Washington and Lee Law Review* 58 (2001): 1427–90.

7. Hyman, "Health Care Fraud" (see note 26, chapter 2); also see Paul E. Kalb, "Fraud and Abuse Law," *Journal of the America Medical Association* 282 (1999): 1163–68.

8. 42 U.S.C. §1320a-7b(b).

9. 42 U.S.C. §1395nn.

10. 31 U.S.C. §3729.

11. *United States v. Krizek*, 111 F.3d 934 (D.C. Cir. 1997).

12. James F. Blumstein, "The Fraud and Abuse Statute in an Evolving Health Care Marketplace: Life in the Health Care Speakeasy," *American Journal of Law and Medicine* 22 (1996): 205, 218.

13. Hyman, "Health Care Fraud" (see note 26, chapter 2).

14. Ibid., p. 550.

15. *United States v. Jain*, 93 F.3d 436 (8th Cir. 1996).

16. *Fraud and Abuse: Do Current Laws Protect the Public Interest?* (Washington: American Health Lawyers Association 1999), p. 10.

17. Hyman, "Health Care Fraud" (see note 26, chapter 2).

18. See, for example, the Clifford Law Offices' Web site on Not-For-Profit Hospital Class Action Litigation: http://www.cliffordlaw.com/not-for-profit-hospital-class-action-litigation.

Chapter 4

1. Jonathan Skinner and John E. Wennberg, "Exceptionalism or Extravagance: What's Different about Health Care in South Florida?" *Health Affairs* W3 (2003): 372–5.

2. C. Eugene Steuerle and Adam Carasso, "Lifetime Social Security and Medicare Benefits," Urban Institute, March 31, 2003, http://www.urban.org/publications/310667.html.

3. Clark C. Havighurst and Barak D. Richman, "Distributive Injustice(s) in American Health Care," *Law and Contemporary Problems* (forthcoming, 2006).

4. Richard Himmelfarb, *Catastrophic Politics: The Rise and Fall of the Medicare Catastrophic Coverage Act of 1988* (University Park: Penn State Press, 1995); Jill Quadagno, *One Nation, Uninsured* (New York: Oxford University Press, 2005), pp.149–59.

5. Himmelfarb, *Catastrophic Politics,* p. 73.

6. Blevins, *Medicare's Midlife Crisis,* p. 22 (see note 7, chapter 2).

7. William Recktenwald, "Insurance Forum Turns Catastrophic for Rostenkowski," *Chicago Tribune,* August 18, 1989, p. 1.

8. Mike Royko, *Chicago Tribune,* August 18, 1989, p. 2.

9. Himmelfarb, *Catastrophic Politics,* p. 82.

10. Ibid., pp. 81–82.

11. Quadagno, *One Nation,* p. 158.

12. Ibid.

13. Himmelfarb, *Catastrophic Politics,* p. 83.

14. Ibid.

15. NBC Broadcast, Aug. 18, 1989

16. Statement of Douglas Holtz-Eakin before the U.S. House of Representatives Committee on Ways and Means, "Prescription Drug Coverage and

Medicare's Fiscal Challenges," Congressional Budget Office, April 9, 2003, p. 9, http://www.cbo.gov/ftpdocs/41xx/doc4159/04-09-PrescriptionDrugs.pdf.

17. Margaret Davis et al., "Prescription Drug Coverage, Utilization, and Spending among Medicare Beneficiaries," *Health Affairs* 18 (Jan.–Feb. 1999): 231.

18. Meredith B. Rosenthal, "Doughnut Hole Economics," *Health Affairs* 23 (Nov.–Dec. 2004): 129, 134.

Chapter 5

1. General Accounting Office, "Medicare Management: CMS Faces Challenges to Sustain Progress and Address Weaknesses," GAO-01-817, p. 2; Stuart M. Butler et al., Open Letter to Congress and the Executive, "Crisis Facing HCFA and Millions of Americans," *Health Affairs* 18 (1999): 8.

2. Marilyn Moon and Christina Boccuti, "Location, Location, Location; Geographic Spending Issues and Medicare Policy," Urban Institute, June 21, 2002, http://www.urban.org/publications/310500.html; Barbara Gage, Marilyn Moon, and Sang Chi, "State-Level Variation in Medicare Spending," *Health Care Financing Review* 85 (Winter 1999): 85–98, http://www.cms.hhs.gov/apps/review/99winter/ 99winterpg85.pdf.

3. See statement of David Glass, "State-Level Variation in Medicare Spending: Preliminary Observations," Medicare Payment Advisory Commission Public Meeting, April 26, 2002, pp. 1–4, http://www.medpac.gov/public_meetings/transcripts/0426_statelevelvariations_DG_transc.pdf.

4. John E. Wennberg, Elliot S. Fisher, and Jonathan Skinner, "Geography and the Debate over Medicare Reform," *Health Affairs Web Exclusive*, February 16, 2002, p. W97, http://content.healthaffairs.org/cgi/reprint/hlthaff.w2. 96v1.pdf; Skinner and Wennberg, "Exceptionalism or Extravagance," pp. 372–5.

5. Dartmouth Atlas of Health Care, visited September 30, 2003, http:// www.dartmouthatlas.org/.

6. See Centers for Medicare and Medicaid Services, "Note to: Medicare and Choice Organizations and Other Interested Parties," May 12, 2003, http://cms.hhs.gov/healthplans/rates/2004/cover.asp.

7. See William M. Sage and Peter Hammer, "Competing on Quality of Care: The Need to Develop a Competition Policy for the Health Care Market,"

University of Michigan Journal of Law Reform 32 (1999): 1069, 1073; "Medicare, Equity and Justice," Minnesota Seniors Federation, 2005, http://mnseniors.org/content/category/3/31/67/.

8. See generally *Minn. Senior Fed'n, Metro. Region v. United States*, 273 F.3d 805 (8th Cir. 2001), cert. denied, 536 U.S. 939 (2002).

9. See "The Geographic Coalition Homepage for a Fair Medicare Reimbursement System," http://www.mnmed.org/images/Gc/index.html.

10. See "Iowa Cares about Medicare Coalition," Medicare Equity in the News, visited September 30, 2003, http://www.iowamedicare.org/news.shtml.

11. See Lieutenant Governor Sally Pederson, "Iowa Deserves a Fair Share of Medicare," July 16, 2002, http://www.governor.state.ia.us/lt_gov/2002/07_16_02.pdf.

12. See Minnesota Medical Association Online, http://www.mmaonline.net/pdf/rollcallad.pdf.

13. Susan Bartlett Foote, "Why Medicare Cannot Promulgate a National Coverage Rule: A Case of Regula Mortis," *Journal of Health Policy, Politics and Law* 27 (2002): 707, 708–20.

Chapter 6

1. Hyman, "Does Quality of Care Matter to Medicare?" (see note 28, chapter 2), pp. 55–68.

2. Marmor, *Politics of Medicare,* p. 97.

3. David Hyman and Mark Hall, "Two Cheers for Employment-Based Health Insurance," *Yale Journal of Health Policy, Law and Ethics* 2 (2001): 23, 35.

4. Hyman, "Does Quality of Care Matter" (see note 28, chapter 2), p. 60.

5. See "From a Generation Behind to a Generation Ahead: Transforming Traditional Medicare," National Academy of Social Insurance Study Panel on Fee-for-Service Medicare, January 1998, http://www.nasi.org/usr_doc/med_report_gen_behind.pdf.

6. Paul Ginsburg, testimony before the Senate Finance Committee, "Comparing the Traditional Medicare Program to Private Insurance," May 12, 1999, http://finance.senate.gov/5-12gins.htm#N_4.

7. See Bryan Dowd et al., "A Tale of Four Cities: Medicare Reform and Competitive Pricing," *Health Affairs* (Sept.–Oct. 2000): 9, 11.

Chapter 7

1. See "In the Case of Blue Shield of California," Medicare Appeals Council, June 20, 2003, http://www.hhs.gov/dab/macdecision/blueshieldca.htm.

2. See Richard A. Epstein, *Mortal Peril* (Boston: Addison Wesley, 1997), pp. 200–202.

3. Nicholas Lemann, "America Right and Left," *The Atlantic Online*, 4, ¶ 27, April 1998, visited August 24, 2003, http://www.theatlantic.com/issues/98apr/leftrite.htm.

4. David Espo, "Parties Debate Medicare, Social Security," Associated Press, June 18, 2002.

5. See Andrew A. Green, "2nd District Debate Features Collegiality, Jabs," *Baltimore Sun*, October 29, 2002, p. 3B.

6. See Dana Milbank, "The Campaign Seasoning: The Flavor of the Week," *Washington Post*, September 30, 2004, p. C4.

7. See Noam Scheiber, "The Old Way," *New Republic*, February 11, 2002, pp. 20–21; Carl M. Cannon, "Medicare Fiscal Woes Accelerate," *Baltimore Sun*, June 6, 1996, p. 1A.

8. See "Reaction to the Second Clinton/Dole Debate," *NewsHour with Jim Lehrer*, PBS Television Broadcast, October 16, 1996, http://www.pbs.org/newshour/debatingourdestiny/newshour/96reax_partisans_10-16.html.

9. See Uwe Reinhardt, "Demagoguery and Debate over Medicare Reform," *Health Affairs* (Winter 1995): 101.

10. See Memorandum from Rich Thau, "Third Millennium to Frank Luntz and Jeffery Pollock," March 14, 2001, http://www.thirdmil.org/publications/surveys/0103medicarefindings.html.

11. See Mona Charen, "The Bumbler Bowls Them Over," *Jewish World Review*, November 8, 2002, http://www.jewishworldreview.com/cols/charen110802.asp.

12. Pear, "Medicare Agency Changes Name," p. A26 (see note 10, chapter 2).

13. David Frum, "Bad Decision, Good Result," *National Post* (Canada), June 14, 2004.

Chapter 8

1. Dick Armey, *Armey's Axioms: 40 Hard-Earned Truths from Politics, Faith, and Life* (Hoboken, NJ: Wiley, 2003).

2. John Iglehart, "The New Medicare Prescription-Drug Benefit—A Pure Power Play," *New England Journal of Medicine* 350 (2004): 826, 832.

3. Nancy Pelosi, "Remarks at Rally of Seniors Opposed to Republican Medicare Bill," November 19, 2003, http://www.democraticwhip.house.gov/docuploads/med_ara.pdf.

4. Nancy Pelosi, "Tactics on Medicare Bill Brought Dishonor to This House," press release, November 22, 2003, http://www.democraticleader.house.gov/press/releases.cfm?pressReleaseID = 387.

5. Ed Markey, "Medicare Rx Debate" *NewsHour with Jim Lehrer,* PBS Television Broadcast, June 27, 2003, http://www.pbs.org/newshour/bb/health/jan-june03/medicare_06-27.html.

6. Iglehart, "New Medicare Prescription-Drug Benefit."

7. David S. Broder, "Time Was GOP's Ally on the Vote," *Washington Post,* November 23, 2003, p. A1.

8. Anthony Beilenson, "Leadership and Politics: Four Views," in *Medicare: Preparing for the Challenges of the 21st Century,* ed. Robert D. Reischauer et al. (Washington: Brookings Institution Press, 1998), pp. 261–3.

Chapter 9

1. P. J. O'Rourke, *Parliament of Whores* (New York: Vintage, 1991), p. 177.

2. Saul Bellow, accessed April 5, 2006, http://www.quotemeonit.com/bellow.html.

Chapter 10

1. Peter Fisher, "Speech to Columbus Council on World Affairs," U.S. Treasury Department, November 14, 2002, http://www.treas.gov/press/releases/po3622.htm.

2. Social Security and Medicare Boards of Trustees, "Status of the Social Security and Medicare Programs; A Summary of the 2006 Annual Reports," May 2, 2006, http://www.ssa.gov/OACT/TRSUM/trsummary.html.

3. Jonathan Oberlander, *The Political Life of Medicare* (Chicago: University of Chicago Press, 2003).

4. Theodore R. Marmor, "How Not to Think about Medicare Reform," *Journal of Health Politics, Policy and Law,* 26 (2001): 107, 113–4.

5. Boards of Trustees, Federal Hospital Insurance and Federal Supplementary Medical Insurance Trust Funds, *2006 Annual Report of the Boards of Trustees of the Federal Hospital Insurance and Federal Supplementary Medical Insurance Trust Funds* (Washington: Government Printing Office, 2006), pp. 65, 105, 116, http://www.cms.hhs.gov/ReportsTrustFunds/downloads/tr2006.pdf.

6. Boards of Trustees, Federal Hospital Insurance and Federal Supplementary Medical Insurance Trust Funds, *2006 Annual Report of the Boards of Trustees of the Federal Hospital Insurance and Federal Supplementary Medical Insurance Trust Funds* (Washington: Government Printing Office, 2006) p. 18, http://www.cms.hhs.gov/ReportsTrustFunds/downloads/tr2006.pdf.

7. Jonathan Cohn, "The Single Guy," *New Republic ¶ 12,* November 22, 2002, http://www/tnr.com/doc.mhtml?i = express/sc = cohn112202.

8. U.S. Office of Management and Budget, *Budget of the United States Government, Fiscal Year 2000: Analytical Perspectives* (Washington: Government Printing Office, 1999), p. 337.

9. Blevins, *Medicare's Midlife Crises,* p. 13 (see note 7, chapter 2).

10. Donna Shalala, Secretary of Health and Human Services, Statement to the House Ways and Means Committee, 105th Congress, 1st session, February 12, 1997, http://waysandmeans.house.gov/Legacy/ fullcomm/105cong/2-12-97/2-12shal.htm and http://commdocs.house.gov/committees/ways/hwmw105-17.000/hwmw105-17_0f.htm.

11. Douglas Holtz-Eakin, "H.R. 1, Medicare Prescription Drug, Improvement, and Modernization Act of 2003," U.S. Congressional Budget Office, November 20, 2003, pp. 1, 8, http://www.cbo.gov/ftpdocs/48xx/ doc4808/11-20-MedicareLetter.pdf.

12. U.S. Office of Management and Budget, "Table S–13. Outlay Impact of Prescription Drug and Medicare Improvement Act of 2003 (P.L. 108-173)," *Budget of the United States Government, Fiscal Year 2005,* February, 2004, p. 387, http://www.whitehouse.gov/omb/budget/fy2005/pdf/budget/tables.pdf.

13. *2004 Annual Report of the Boards of Trustees of the Federal Hospital Insurance and Federal Supplementary Medical Insurance Trust Funds,* March

23, 2004, Table IV.F5, p. 190, cited in Joseph Antos and Jagadeesh Gokhale, "Medicare Prescription Drugs: Medical Necessity Meets Fiscal Insanity," Cato Institute Briefing Paper no. 91, February 9, 2005, p. 9, http://www.cato.org/pubs/briefs/bp91.pdf.

14. Bush administration budget estimate for September 2004, cited in Antos and Gokhale, "Medicare Prescription Drugs," p. 3.

15. Bush administration budget estimate for September, 2005, cited in Antos and Gokhale, "Medicare Prescription Drugs," p. 3.

Chapter 11

1. Jonathan Rauch, "Good Idea GOPers—But It Didn't Work in Britain," *Jewish World Review,* December 23, 2004, http://www.jewishworldreview.com/jonathan/rauch1.asp. See also http://www.cato.org/special/_ownership_society/index.html.

2. Fred Barnes, "We Are What We Own," *The Opinion Journal Online,* from the *Wall Street Journal* editorial page, January 31, 2006, http://www.opinionjournal.com/editorial/feature.html?id = 110007900.

3. John S. Hoff, *Medicare Private Contracting: Paternalism or Autonomy* (Washington: American Enterprise Institute, 1998).

4. Janice A. Hauge, "Contradictory Incentives in the Medicare + Choice Medical Savings Account Program," *Cato Journal* 26 (Winter 2006):125-142.

5. U.S. Federal Trade Commission and U.S. Department of Justice, *Improving Health Care: A Dose of Competition,* July 2004, http://www.usdoj.gov/atr/public/health_care/204694.htm.

6. Frank H. Easterbrook, "Contract and Copyright," *Houston Law Review* 42, no. 4. (Symposium 2005): 967, http://www.houstonlawreview.org/archive/downloads/42-4_pdf/Easterbrook.pdf.

7. Thomas Scully, Commentary in *Medicare: Preparing for the Challenges of the 21st Century,* ed. Robert D. Reischauer et al. (Washington: Brookings Institution Press, 1997).

8. Reinhardt, "Demagoguery and Debate," p. 101 (see note 9, chapter 7).

9. Albert J. Dunlap, *Mean Business: How I Save Bad Companies and Make Good Companies Great,* 1st ed. (New York: Crown Business, 1996), p. 48.

Chapter 12

1. *The Usual Suspects,* Gramercy Pictures, 1995.

2. See Theda Skocpol, *Boomerang: Clinton's Health Security Effort and the Turn against Government in U.S. Politics* (New York: W. W. Norton, 1996).

3. Robert D. Putnam et al., *Making Democracy Work: Civic Traditions in Modern Italy,* 1st ed. (Princeton, NJ: Princeton University Press, 1993), p. 177.

Chapter 13

1. Elizabeth S. Kubler-Ross, *On Death and Dying* (New York: Macmillan Publishing, 1969).

2. Milton Friedman, "Remarks at White House Ceremony in His Honor, May 9, 2002," *Cato Institute Policy Report,* no. 11, http://www.cato.org/pubs/policy-report/v24n4/change-history.pdf. President Bush's remarks on the occasion may be found at http://www.whitehouse.gov/news/releases/2002/05/20020509-1.html.

3. *Austin Powers: International Man of Mystery,* New Line Cinema, 1997.

4. Herbert Stein, "Herb Stein's Unfamiliar Quotations," *Slate.com,* May 16, 1997, http://www.slate.com/id/2561/.

Index

About the Author

David A. Hyman is a professor of law and medicine at the University of Illinois and an adjunct scholar at the Cato Institute. He served as a Special Counsel at the U.S. Federal Trade Commission from November 2001 through November 2004. He was the principal author of the first joint report ever issued by the Federal Trade Commission and the Department of Justice, titled *Improving Health Care: A Dose of Competition.* He has published articles in law reviews, medical journals, and peer-reviewed policy journals on a variety of issues involving health care financing and regulation. He lives in Champaign, Illinois.

Cato Institute

Founded in 1977, the Cato Institute is a public policy research foundation dedicated to broadening the parameters of policy debate to allow consideration of more options that are consistent with the traditional American principles of limited government, individual liberty, and peace. To that end, the Institute strives to achieve greater involvement of the intelligent, concerned lay public in questions of policy and the proper role of government.

The Institute is named for *Cato's Letters,* libertarian pamphlets that were widely read in the American Colonies in the early 18th century and played a major role in laying the philosophical foundation for the American Revolution.

Despite the achievement of the nation's Founders, today virtually no aspect of life is free from government encroachment. A pervasive intolerance for individual rights is shown by government's arbitrary intrusions into private economic transactions and its disregard for civil liberties.

To counter that trend, the Cato Institute undertakes an extensive publications program that addresses the complete spectrum of policy issues. Books, monographs, and shorter studies are commissioned to examine the federal budget, Social Security, regulation, military spending, international trade, and myriad other issues. Major policy conferences are held throughout the year, from which papers are published thrice yearly in the *Cato Journal.* The Institute also publishes the quarterly magazine *Regulation.*

In order to maintain its independence, the Cato Institute accepts no government funding. Contributions are received from foundations, corporations, and individuals, and other revenue is generated from the sale of publications. The Institute is a nonprofit, tax-exempt, educational foundation under Section 501(c)3 of the Internal Revenue Code.

CATO INSTITUTE
1000 Massachusetts Ave., N.W.
Washington, D.C. 20001
www.cato.org